Pharmaceutical Care Made Easy

Pharmaceutical Care Made Easy

Essentials of medicines management in the individual patient

John Sexton

BPharm(Hons), MSc, MCPP, DipClinPharm, PgCertEd(Teaching and Learning in HE), MRPharmS

Principal Pharmacist Lecturer–Practitioner
Royal Liverpool and Broadgreen University Hospitals NHS Trust,
and Liverpool John Moores University, UK

Gareth Nickless

BPharm(Hons), DipClinPharm, MRPharmS

Senior Pharmacist Clinical Tutor
Royal Liverpool and Broadgreen University Hospitals NHS Trust, UK

Chris Green

BSc(Hons), DipClinPharm, PhD, MRPharmS

Director of Pharmacy and Medicines Management
Countess of Chester Hospital NHS Foundation Trust and Honorary Lecturer,
Liverpool John Moores University, UK

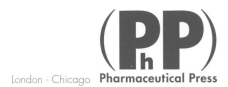

London · Chicago **Pharmaceutical Press**

Published by the Pharmaceutical Press
An imprint of RPS Publishing

1 Lambeth High Street, London SE1 7JN, UK
100 South Atkinson Road, Suite 206, Grayslake, IL 60030-7820, USA

© Pharmaceutical Press 2006

(**PP**)is a trade mark of RPS Publishing

RPS Publishing is the publishing organisation of the Royal Pharmaceutical Society of Great Britain

First published 2006

Typeset by J&L Composition, Filey, North Yorkshire
Printed in Great Britain by Cambridge University Press, Cambridge

ISBN-10 0 85369 650 0
ISBN-13 978 0 85369 650 6

A catalogue record for this book is available from the British Library

This book is dedicated to all the colleagues, students and patients we have encountered over the years whose contribution to our practice can never be quantified

All the authors' royalties from the preparation of this book are to be donated to charity.

Contents

Section 3: Examples of Pharmaceutical Care Planning   159

Preface

Students of pharmacy, preregistration graduates, pharmacists and pharmacy technicians are faced with the same challenge every time they come into contact with a patient – how to provide effective care, pharmaceutical care, which will deliver improved outcomes to the patient. Patients are increasingly presenting with prescriptions that a decade ago would have been labelled as polypharmaceutical, especially where there is substantial co-morbidity. In recent years publications such as *A Spoonful of Sugar* and *An Organisation with a Memory* have highlighted the likely rates of drug-induced harm in patient care.[1,2] Hepler and Strand had already proclaimed in 1990 that, 'if the public knew that which pharmacists did about drug-related morbidity and mortality, they would not just allow pharmacists to practice pharmaceutical care, they would demand it'.[3]

It is the view of the authors of this book that few patients' therapies need intimidate even the generalist or student. We remain ever more convinced that clear thought processes can bring order to even seemingly complex regimes. It is widely believed that problems should be broken down to their simplest components, to be dealt with systematically. Our clinical colleagues and tutors taught us how to apply that to patient care, and we are mindful of our debt to the thousands of students and patients who have challenged us, inspired us and never ceased to surprise us – often picking up points that had escaped the practitioner at the bedside.

This is not a textbook of therapeutics – other sources to which we refer constantly do this much better, with each chapter written by expert practitioners in that field. This is not even a detailed guide to the theoretical models of pharmaceutical care – wiser minds than ours have described these well in a series of articles and books over the last two decades. But it is a book for those who want to improve their practice, bring clarity and order to drug regimes, and contribute to patients' care. This book does not consider the specific care of the paediatric patient, and although many of the principles are applicable to paediatrics, that particular work is still awaited from the specialists in that area of practice. The therapeutic pathways that we describe are not the only suitable ones, and may well change as evidence bases grow. They do, however, describe the consensus of best practice in the experience of local colleagues, correspond with the most recent NHS and professional guidance, and illustrate how to pick a path through the multitude of choices available to pharmacists and prescribers. We are also pleased not only to link our pathways with the most recent guidance, but also to guide the reader to the suitable online background reading available in each condition. As such, references are kept to a minimum. All online material, indicated in the text by '(ONLINE)', can be accessed quickly through the associated website: www.pharmpress.com/onlineresources

We wish you every success in your endeavours!

References

1 Audit Commission. *A Spoonful of Sugar – medicines management in NHS hospitals*. London: Audit Commission; 2001. (ONLINE)

2 Department of Health. *An Organisation with a Memory*. Report of an expert working group on learning from adverse events in the NHS chaired by the Chief Medical Officer. London: The Stationery Office; 2000. (ONLINE)

3 Hepler C, Strand L. Opportunities and responsibilities in pharmaceutical care. *Am J Hosp Pharm* 1990; 47: 533–543.

About the authors

John Sexton, BPharm(Hons), MSc, MCPP, DipClinPharm, PgCert Ed, MRPharmS, is Principal Pharmacist Lecturer–Practitioner at the Royal Liverpool and Broadgreen University Hospitals NHS Trust and Liverpool John Moores University. His NHS role is as directorate pharmacist for nephrology and transplantation, and at Liverpool John Moores University he leads the teaching of clinical pharmacy and therapeutics.

Gareth Nickless, BPharm(Hons), DipClinPharm, MRPharmS, is Senior Pharmacist Clinical Tutor at the Royal Liverpool and Broadgreen University Hospitals NHS Trust. His NHS role is as directorate pharmacist to gastroenterology, and he contributes to both bedside and university teaching of undergraduate and postgraduate students.

Chris Green, BSc(Hons), DipClinPharm, PhD, MRPharmS, is Director of Pharmacy and Medicines Management at the Countess of Chester Hospital NHS Foundation Trust and an Honorary Lecturer at Liverpool John Moores University. He has been actively involved in pharmaceutical education and professional development over many years.

The authors collectively have over 20 years' experience in teaching clinical pharmacy in both academic and clinical environments to undergraduates and postgraduates. This book has its roots in a successful undergraduate module at Liverpool John Moores University, 'Clinical pharmacy and therapeutics'. Many pharmacists have been responsible for the development of this module and its continual refinement and improvement over two decades, and continue to participate in its delivery to this day.[1]

Reference

1 Caldwell N, Sexton J, Green CF, Farrar K. Sowing the seeds of pharmaceutical care: developments in undergraduate clinical teaching at Liverpool School of Pharmacy. *Pharm J* 2001; **267**: 721–723. (ONLINE)

Further reading

The therapeutics sections in this book refer frequently to four standard texts, familiar to students and practitioners. These are listed below:

- *British National Formulary*, 51st edn. London: British Medical Association and Royal Pharmaceutical Society of Great Britain; 2006. (£22.95/ISBN 085369 668 3) The essential companion of every student and practitioner of pharmaceutical care.

- Dodds LJ. *Drugs in Use*, 3rd edn. London: Pharmaceutical Press; 2003. (£29.95/ISBN 085369 541 5) For the preregistration graduate and working pharmacist – a series of practical cases to work through.

- Randall MD, Neil KE. *Disease Management*. London: Pharmaceutical Press; 2004. (£29.95/ISBN 085369 523 7) A basic introduction to disease states and their management for the undergraduate or technical student.

- Walker R, Edwards CRW. *Clinical Pharmacy and Therapeutics*, 3rd edn. London: Churchill-Livingstone; 2003. (£41.99/ISBN 044307 137 3) An invaluable introduction to disease states and their management for the undergraduate or technical student.

Section 1

The Basics of Pharmaceutical Care

1. CONCENTRATE: It's not rocket science!

Don't be intimidated by a patient's problems. Most of the problems that lead to morbidity and mortality can be spotted by a thorough approach. In the high-profile reports of serious harm occurring to a patient, usually something simple (though serious) has gone wrong.

2. SEARCH: What are the problems?

The basis of pharmaceutical care is a thorough identification of all of a patient's actual and potential medical conditions and other relevant problems (e.g. devices, compliance or difficulties in obtaining supplies). The problem list is assembled from all the available information, and prioritised in terms of urgency for action.

We discuss this in:

Problem identification and prioritisation

3. DECIDE + ACT: What needs to be done about each problem?

For each problem, a solution will present itself. It may be that no therapy requires starting, stopping or changing, but if a change to current therapy is indicated then the alternative approaches should be considered, an appropriate choice recommended and a suitable initiating dose decided upon. In any event, appropriate monitoring is essential to ensure efficacy and safety of any therapy.

We discuss this in:

Problem handling

Introduction: what is pharmaceutical care?

Pharmacists were traditionally experts in drugs. In about 200 BC, the Jewish prophet Sirach wrote that 'the pharmacist mixes these medicines, and the doctor then uses them to cure diseases and ease pain'. This encapsulates a traditional view of the pharmacist's role that did not begin to change until the 1970s. At that time, in the US and in British hospitals, pharmacists began to leave their dispensaries to engage in ward pharmacy, which later developed into clinical pharmacy. Complementary developments also occurred in the roles of community pharmacists and technical staff. Specialist pharmaceutical knowledge and skills were contributing to patient care to deliver drug therapy that was safe, effective and cost-effective.

In 1990, in one of the most cited papers in the pharmaceutical literature, Douglas Hepler and Linda Strand defined a philosophy of pharmaceutical care, based around the identification, resolution and prevention of drug-related problems, to reduce mortality (premature death) and morbidity (ill-health) caused by poorly or inadequately applied drug therapy.[1] However, a variety of problems with the application of this theory led to its development, in conjunction with other practitioners, into a practice of pharmaceutical care, which was defined as 'a practice in which the practitioner takes responsibility for a patient's drug-related needs, and is held accountable for this commitment'.[2,3] In a practice model, familiar to other professions and healthcare professionals, and equally applicable to primary and secondary care, three essential stages were defined: the assessment, a care plan and an evaluation, succeeded by continuous follow-up.

In this book, this definition of pharmaceutical care is not overturned, but a slightly different approach is proposed. An over-reliance on the term 'drug-related problem' is avoided by substitution with the broader idea of the 'pharmaceutical care problem', which we define on p. 4. A model is illustrated for assessing the newly admitted hospital patient, or the patient being engaged in a medication review exercise in primary care, and a holistic approach to their care to improve their quality of life is taken. This model has two stages:

1. Identification of all the medical and pharmaceutical problems that a patient has and assembly into a list in order of priority for action or otherwise by the pharmaceutical care provider.
2. Handling of each problem individually, assessment of whether the aims of therapy are being met, application of therapeutic guidelines to decide what action is needed, and the implementation and monitoring of this action.

The need for continuous follow-up outlined by the successors to Hepler and Strand makes this process cyclical and defines our process for handling each problem as summarised in Figure 1.1.[1]

Pharmaceutical care or medicines management?

In this book we use the term 'pharmaceutical care' to describe how pharmacists can contribute to the achievement of desired therapeutic outcomes in patient care, reducing morbidity and mortality. Some British pharmacists are unhappy to use a term that has become closely identified with a particular model of practice, as applied in an overseas

Figure 1.1 The pharmaceutical care cycle

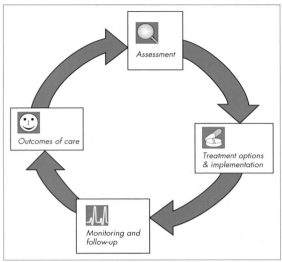

Assessment

Treatment options
& implementation

Monitoring and
follow-up

Outcomes of care

health system. The term 'medicines management' has become popular in recent NHS documents, and has gained favour in the UK among pharmacy managers because it is clearly advantageous to use a terminology that other professions and NHS managers can understand. Medicines management encompasses all the activities that contribute to safe and rational medicines use, including strategic functions such as purchasing, formulary policy, risk management and many other roles of pharmacists and pharmacy technicians. However, it clearly includes the application of pharmaceutical knowledge and skills to the individual patient, though some would argue that medicines management does not demand the full role and patient responsibility demanded by the standard works on pharmaceutical care – the controversy was aired in 2001.[4] Whichever term is used, all agree with the 1990 call of Hepler and Strand for pharmacists to accept their responsibility to deliver effective and safe patient care and improve the quality of life of their patients.[1]

PI Problem identification and prioritisation

In this book the term 'problem' means pharmaceutical care problem. A pharmaceutical care problem can be defined as in the box below.

A pharmaceutical care problem is any medical or patient problem that can be:
- cured
- ameliorated (helped, made better)
- prevented
- caused
- aggravated
- or affected in any other way

by either:
- drug therapy

or
- the application of pharmaceutical skills or knowledge.

PI1: What is a problem?

Once the relationship with the patient has been established, pharmaceutical care begins with the construction of a problem list and prioritisation of its contents. The first (and most important) question that should be asked when constructing a pharmaceutical care plan is 'What are the patient's problems?'.

Pharmacists might consider a patient's problems in one of two ways, classifying them by either their derivation or their existence, as detailed below.

Derivation: medical and pharmaceutical problems

Medical problems describe the disease states that the patient may be suffering from, such as Crohn's disease, asthma or an adverse drug reaction. Referral letters, 'clerking-in' notes made by a doctor or nurse-practitioner, or medical records in primary care are all useful initial sources of this information. Over-reliance on these sources should, however, be avoided. For example, a doctor admitting a patient into hospital may not have access to all the information needed to assemble a complete problem list or may be working in a situation in which they are focusing on the immediate problem in hand.

Pharmaceutical problems relate to issues arising from the delivery of drug therapy and may not be considered by the physician in their initial assessment of the patient. Examples include difficulty using inhalers, polypharmacy resulting in poor compliance, and so forth. A good pharmacist takes a broader view of patients than their medical problems and prescription. They should be able to review the patient with a consideration of the problems that may result from drug therapy, and apply a particular focus on how the individual patient will manage and take his or her medicines.

Existence: actual and potential problems

Actual problems are problems that the patient is currently experiencing, even if they are well controlled. For example, they may have ischaemic heart disease or, on testing, display poor inhaler technique.

Potential problems are those that the patient is not currently experiencing but is at risk of developing due to either drug therapy prescribed or concurrent disease states. Examples might include the risk of developing osteoporosis if a patient is prescribed long-term corticosteroid therapy, or the chance of developing cardiovascular disease in a hypertensive patient.

The inter-relationship of actual, potential, medical and pharmaceutical problems is described in Table 1.1. It should be noted that a patient might have problems from one, several or all of these groups.

Remember

There is no precise way of defining the scope of each pharmaceutical care problem identified. A good example of this is seen in **Nephrology N2**: The patient has severe chronic kidney disease. The problem is considered as a whole, as defined in the chapter title, rather than using a chapter in this book for each parameter or subproblem commonly associated with severe renal failure. These parameters are instead considered as the subproblems of renal failure. However, a specialist renal pharmacist might look at each as a problem in its own right.

Table 1.1 The classification of pharmaceutical care problems by derivation and existence

Actual problems	Potential problems
Actual medical problems: e.g. patient has hypertension, asthma	**Potential medical problems**: e.g. risk of cardiovascular disease in a hypertensive patient, risk of gastrointestinal bleed in a patient prescribed long-term non-steroidal anti-inflammatory drug (NSAID) therapy
Actual pharmaceutical problems: e.g. the patient exhibits poor inhaler technique	**Potential pharmaceutical problems**: e.g. concordance issues, compliance problems, education needs, effects of confusion in elderly patients, difficulty in obtaining supplies

PI2: Identifying the problems

A variety of methods may be used to identify an individual patient's problems. Much of the information is easily available – it just has to be gathered.

Figure 1.2 shows the most common sources used to derive the current problem list and prioritise it. These might seem onerous, but in practice can be reviewed quite quickly. As a minimum we would imagine that most newly admitted hospital patients (or patients being reviewed in the community) would have the following sources reviewed on admission or review:

- the medication history (with action taken if there are omissions and errors)
- a set of basic relevant blood results
- the initial inpatient prescription chart (if a hospital admission) or current drug record (in primary care)
- a quick review of the case-notes to establish the reason for admission or request for review, along with any significant concurrent disease states (co-morbidity)
- a conversation with the patient if at all possible (and/or their carers, if appropriate) to confirm all the above and establish any extra information needed.

The impression the pharmacist gains while looking at and speaking with the patient should not be underestimated. An intuition, developed with experience, will help indicate factors that deserve further attention.

PI3: The medication history and patient interview

An important source of information in the initial assessment is the medication history. This is a record of the drugs that a patient is taking at the time of admission/review and is a key part of a medication review and of hospital admission processes in many NHS trusts. Although it is called a history, in general, previous medication and durations of therapy are of secondary importance unless adverse events/drug sensitivities/treatment

Figure 1.2 Common sources for deriving the problem list

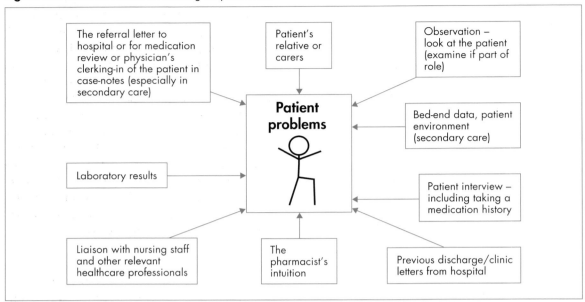

failures were associated with the therapy, or the treatment is only newly started. Other than the patient and any information they keep themselves, the information sources that may initially be available are shown in Box 1.1.

Process

Not all the sources of information will be readily available to you during the initial assessment, nor is it appropriate to use them all initially. Remember, no single source of information can always be completely trusted – much recent research has shown that medical records and letters are full of omissions, errors and ambiguities, to an extent that would horrify most patients. After briefly reviewing the information readily available to you, you are ready to talk to the patient, whom you expect to be your major source of verifiable information. If this is not possible, or does not deliver sufficient information, it may be necessary to revisit some of the sources not yet utilised, and secondary care practitioners may need to telephone general practitioner (GP) surgeries or community pharmacies.

Pharmacist-acquired medication histories are especially important on hospital admission because the quality of information recorded in case-notes (especially during clerking-in) varies widely. This may be because the junior medical staff do not have access to all the information needed themselves or because patients become nervous or lie to avoid offending or disappointing the doctor. In addition, the pharmacist can bring specialist knowledge to bear about brands, formulations, unusual products and possible relationships between drug therapy and medical problems or essential monitoring.

The patient interview: principles

Partnership

Occasionally a patient on multiple long-term drug therapy will present motivated, lucid and with a meticulously maintained self-managed list of their medication. Medication histories will be easy to clarify in this type of patient. Many more will be unable to remember facts, and while gentle encouragement is appropriate to encourage co-responsibility for managing medication and

Box 1.1 Potential initial information sources

- **Medication** brought in to the hospital/surgery or seen in the domiciliary situation ('brown-bag' review) *but* remember that:
  — just because it is there does not mean that the patient has been taking it or is taking it exactly as intended
  — labels may no longer be correct; 'Doctor said to double up on that one', or may not be available if tablets have been removed from original packs
  — have you seen everything that the patient is taking? Don't forget to check for over-the-counter drugs (OTCs)/herbal medicines/insulins etc. Patients may not immediately associate these with the term 'medicines'
- **FP10 copies** may be available – many patients carry these around with them *or* hospital pharmacists can ask GP surgeries to fax over a copy of current medication *but*:
  — these records can be wrong, incomplete or out of date even in the best GP practices
  — again, just because the GP thinks that the patient is taking it, doesn't mean that they are
  — data can be incomplete, e.g. 'As directed', 'Two daily'
  — no OTCs or medication provided by other sources (e.g. trials, homecare schemes) will be listed
- **Community pharmacists (if the patient is loyal to one)/recent hospital discharge** information may be available *but*:
  — is it complete?
  — is it up to date?
  — does the patient actually take that which is dispensed?
- **Patient records/case-notes** may contain information about drug therapy, reason for admission, and so forth, but have similar limitations to the above sources. Medical records are often incomplete or inaccurate
- **Medical/nursing staff** in the ward/surgery situation or **administration records from nursing homes** and the **information provided by relatives or carers** may additionally throw light on the drug history, reason for admission and additional drug-related problems

avoiding reliance on professionals to do this, you are not the patient's judge. Remember that they may be elderly, anxious about their interview or admission to hospital, acutely unwell, confused or simply unable to remember long lists of drugs with strengths and frequencies of dosing.

Sensitivity

Good practice requires that pharmacists, technicians, doctors and nurses not only introduce themselves, but ask a few conversational questions first (unless circumstances render this inappropriate). This not only relaxes the patient, which will improve clarity of thought and recall, but establishes whether the patient is fit to be interviewed at that point in time. The focus can then be narrowed with questions such as, 'Right, Mrs Brown, can we think about your medicines now?'. Similarly, questions about adverse events/non-compliance will elicit more honest answers if the patient trusts the pharmacist enough not to feel the need to evade or lie. This can be encouraged by asking non-judgemental questions such as: 'A lot of people would struggle to remember to take all those, Mr. White, does that ever happen to you?'

Thoroughness

If the patient has brought medication or a list, use that as a focus for the discussion. Don't forget to ask about recent changes/adverse events/administration problems/drug sensitivities/OTC and herbal medication. Remember that they may forget to include eye drops/inhalers/injections etc. as 'medicines'. The patient should be doing most of the talking if you wish to avoid the errors of an unclear or muddled patient simply agreeing with you. You can then decide which other sources of information may be appropriate to follow-up. A structured form may guide inexperienced staff.

Responsibility

The first responsibility of a pharmacist is to their patient. If you are unsure how much depth it is necessary to go into, imagine that the patient were a relative of yours and what would usually shape your decision. Healthcare professionals have a responsibility to see the patient holistically, as a complete individual, and not as a presenting complaint or a collection of problems, illustrated by comments such as, 'How's the angina patient coming along?'. In addition, no matter how stressed, a pharmacist should never see the patient as a unit of work or a burden. The views of the patient are important and should not be dismissed as irrational or ill-informed, no matter how unorthodox they might appear.

PI4: Initial laboratory tests

Upon initial assessment, the most significant laboratory tests should be reviewed quickly (Table 1.2). Remember that reference ranges vary slightly between laboratories and slight abnormalities may be irrelevant or even perfectly normal in a patient. Changes over time, and trends, may often be as important as actual values.

Other laboratory tests

These are not always available for every newly admitted or reviewed patient, but may have been requested if thought relevant. Some may need to be requested to assess a problem or to ensure that drug therapy is both safe and effective (Table 1.3).

Table 1.2 Initial laboratory tests

Test and typical levels	Usefulness
Na$^+$ (135–145 mmol/L)	Major extracellular ion, wide range means that small changes are often uninterpretable and usually insignificant *High*: dehydration, diabetic ketoacidosis or hyperosmolar coma *Low*: overhydration, SIADH (inappropriate antidiuretic hormone) diuretics (especially combinations), antidepressants, antiepileptics
K$^+$ (3.5–5.5 mmol/L)	Major intracellular ion but narrow range means small changes are important – can cause cardiac arrhythmias *High*: renal failure, diabetic ketoacidosis or hyperosmolar coma (initially), potassium-sparing diuretics, angiotensin-converting enzyme (ACE) inhibitors, angiotensin II receptor antagonists Low: thiazide and loop diuretics, beta-agonists, diarrhoea, vomiting
Creatinine (<110 mmol/L)	Product of muscle turnover, and the best endogenous reflector of renal function *High*: may indicate renal impairment but beware partial interpretation or misinterpretation of serum creatinine (see Nephrology 1)
Urea (<7.5 mmol/L)	Another marker of renal function but more likely to be affected by other conditions, especially hydration status *High*: renal impairment, dehydration, upper gastrointestinal bleed, infections *Low*: poor nutrition, fluid overload
Ca^{2+} (2.2–2.6 mmol/L)	Most calcium in the body is stored in bone but the free portion in plasma is important for muscle function (including cardiac muscle). Make sure that the value has been adjusted for albumin levels, the so-called 'corrected' or 'adjusted' calcium *High*: immobility, too much vitamin D, malignancy, hyperparathyroidism *Low*: vitamin D deficiency/renal failure, hypoparathyroidism
HCO$_3^-$ (22–31 mmol/L)	Major buffer in blood *High*: alkalosis *Low*: acidosis – often seen in severe renal failure
Haemoglobin (Hb) (12–16 g/dL)	Reference range depends on age and sex *Low*: may reflect nutrition, iron status, haemorrhage, chronic gastrointestinal subclinical bleeding Any abnormality should be followed up by looking at the other haematological/iron results

Table 1.3 Other laboratory tests (may be included in initial screen if considered relevant)

Test	Usefulness
Thyroid function tests	Thyroid-stimulating hormone (TSH) and free thyroxine (T_4) will indicate abnormality, often presenting as another medical problem such as confusion or tachycardia
Liver function tests	Much less quantitative than indicators of renal impairment, bilirubin and liver enzymes such as transaminases and gamma-glutamyl transferase indicate liver disorders. Whether this is due to infection, carcinoma, alcoholism or a drug (many possibilities) requires further consideration and intervention (see Gastroenterology 4)
Cardiac enzymes	Older tests such as lactate dehydrogenase and alkaline phosphatase have been superseded by more specific enzymes such as troponin-T. The presence of these in the circulation at a point several hours after chest pain indicates the ischaemic muscle damage typical of a myocardial infarction. Borderline results may be due to acute coronary syndromes (unstable angina/non-Q-wave myocardial infarction (NSTEMI))
Lipids	Serum cholesterol and low-density lipoprotein (LDL)-cholesterol are performed in most patients at some stage: fasting cholesterol should ideally be below 4–5 mmol/L and tightly controlled where there is raised cardiovascular risk (see **Cardiology 4**)
Clotting	Patients on oral anticoagulants or with liver disorders will have an international normalised ratio (INR) performed. In simple terms, an INR of 2 indicates that blood is taking twice as long to clot as the reference standard. This would usually be the minimum effective INR in warfarin therapy for venous thromboembolism, but an indicator of problems in liver disease. Heparin therapy requires different tests
Therapeutic drug levels	See **Pharmaceutical problems 2** – most levels taken are wasted because they cannot be trusted or because they were not required
Full blood count (FBC)	Abnormal white cell count (WCC) or platelets may aid diagnosis

PI5: Initial assessment and prioritisation of problems

The next step is to assess and prioritise the patient's problems. This is a two-part process, as described in Figure 1.3.

Figure 1.3 Initial assessment of the patient's problems

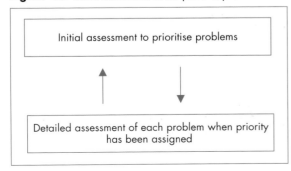

A basic initial assessment of each problem, which identifies severity and whether the problem is active or controlled, aids the prioritisation of problems. This initial assessment involves asking whether the aims of treatment of each problem are being met (e.g. target blood pressure, pain control). An in-depth assessment of each problem can be made after the problems have been prioritised, as described in **Problem handling PH3**. A patient's problems can usually be prioritised as shown in Figure 1.4.

Over the course of time, the priority of each problem may change depending on any response to treatment given. The contents of the problem list may also change – after hospital admission, for example, problems such as chest infections and hypokalaemia may resolve, but new problems may arise (e.g. *Clostridium difficile* diarrhoea).

Figure 1.4 Prioritisation of the patient's problems

Highest priority

The presenting complaint or reason for review is given highest priority since that will have led to the admission or request for review. It must be remembered that the presenting complaint may consist of more than one problem – e.g. a patient with acute renal impairment due to sepsis – and that both of these should be considered as being of the highest priority. However, it is worth noting that, if a patient visits a healthcare professional for an annual medication review, then they will not necessarily have a presenting complaint.

High priority

These are problems where the aims of treatment are not being met and could harm the patient if not resolved immediately. They may be actual or potential and medical or pharmaceutical, e.g. pneumonia requiring antibiotic therapy, uncontrolled hypertension, hyperkalaemia.

Medium priority

These are also problems where the aims of treatment are not being met, but are less likely to cause immediate harm to the patient, e.g. a patient requiring statin therapy for primary prevention, a patient commenced on long-term corticosteroid therapy requiring osteoporosis prophylaxis.

Lowest priority

These are problems where the aims of treatment are being met and will require only continuation of therapy (or no therapy) and routine monitoring, e.g. a patient prescribed allopurinol for prophylaxis of gout who hasn't had an attack for several years.

At the end of the initial assessment you should be in possession of:
- an accurate current medication list
- a prioritised list of the patient's problems
- an awareness of the further information needed and how to get it.

Of course, if you have identified any transcription errors on hospital admission or major errors in the medication record these need correcting (if appropriate) before moving into the second stage of pharmaceutical care – handing each problem individually.

PH Problem handling

PH1: Introduction

Now is the moment to handle each problem individually, starting with the highest-priority problem. The stages are shown in Box 1.2.

These stages are summarised in Figure 1.5. Pharmaceutical care is a cyclical process and the problem, as well as the patient, needs periodic reassessment.

 ## PH2: Defining the desired outcome

'*Would you tell me, please, which way I ought to go from here?*'
'*That depends a good deal on where you want to get to,*' said the Cat.

> Lewis Carroll: Alice's Adventures in Wonderland; 1865

Box 1.2

 Define desired outcomes (PH2)

The desired outcomes of care may be qualitative (e.g. resolution of a rash, absence of pain) or quantitative (e.g. target blood pressure, target haemoglobin). For some medical conditions the aims are set by national bodies or government, e.g. the National Institute for Health and Clinical Excellence (NICE), British Hypertension Society (BHS), National Service Frameworks (NSFs).

 Detailed assessment of each problem (PH3)

While the initial assessment allows priority to be assigned to each problem, the detailed assessment considers the nature and severity of each problem. In addition, the effect of co-morbidities and other current treatment is also considered **(Problem handling PH4)**

 Treatment options (PH5) and implementation (PH6)

In the light of the assessment of how well the current treatment is meeting the desired outcomes of therapy and the options available, the necessary changes can be chosen and made.

 Monitoring (PH7)

The monitoring of safety and efficacy is required to ensure that the outcomes are realised. Reassessment of the problems may well be necessary in light of this.

For every pharmaceutical care problem in your prioritised problem list, there *must* be at least one (and sometimes more than one) desired outcome. Without an outcome there will be no way of knowing if your pharmacotherapeutic interventions are achieving anything.

Figure 1.5 The pharmaceutical care cycle

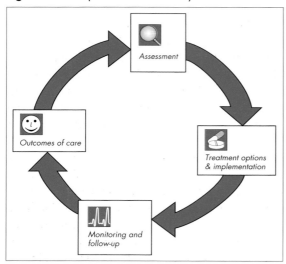

Quantitative and qualitative measures of outcome

Outcomes may be defined using both qualitative and quantitative measures. Quantitative measures are those that can be expressed numerically, such as blood pressure. Qualitative measures are more observational, such as whether or not the patient is vomiting or in pain. Many qualitative observations can be expressed quantitatively, however, such as expressing how many times a patient has vomited, or using numerical scoring systems to assess pain control. This is useful but it is not intended to replace the importance of qualitative assessment. Doctors often say that the first thing they look for when meeting a patient is whether the patient looks well or ill.

Obvious outcomes

If the problem is that the patient is vomiting, the primary desired outcome will be that the patient does not vomit. (And of course this outcome may be only partially achieved, at least initially, but this does not invalidate it as your desired goal). A less obvious desired outcome in this example might be that the anti-emetic therapy does not cause seda-tion, extrapyramidal side-effects or other adverse events.

If the problem is that the patient is non-compliant, then the desired outcome might be that the patient takes all their medication without fail. Again, as with any problem this might not be totally achieved, but, if not, it is time to reassess the patient and try again.

Evidence-based outcomes

In the management of conditions such as hypertension, the obvious outcome is that blood pressure is reduced without causing adverse events. However, the rise of evidence-based medicine (EBM) has led to the defining of target blood pressures and preferred drug choices, proven in large-scale clinical trials to reduce complications such as cardiovascular disease. These targets should inform treatment, but not at the expense of consideration of the patient as an individual, since these trials do not inform how individual patients will respond to any therapy options. Similar issues apply to many chronic conditions.

Changing quantitative measures

With the rise of EBM, especially in cardiovascular disease, there are a number of targets for blood pressure, blood lipids and glucose, and so forth. The targets are set because it is known that, in large trials, people who achieved these targets *on the whole* lived longer, or had fewer complications or fewer hospitalisations. They were, however, sometimes achieved only at the cost of impairing the patients' quality of life with adverse events. As new evidence emerges, targets change, often very rapidly, or different organisations provide different guidance intended for different audiences. So, for instance, many lipid guidelines seek to reduce cholesterol to ≤5 mmol/L, but the most recent British Hypertension Society (BHS) guidance in 2004 (see **Cardiology C4**) seeks ≤4 mmol/L. In a similar manner, the National Institute for Health and Clinical Excellence (NICE) guidance on managing hypertension in primary care (see **Cardiology C1**) suggests more traditional drug choices than these BHS guidelines. In each case, the same evidence is being used, but different judgements are drawn when balancing benefit against risks and economic costs.

The law of diminishing returns

This law states that as more effort is applied to a problem, the incremental improvements or results grow less. Similarly, it is the nature of drug therapy that the first reduction in, for example, serum cholesterol or pain is easier to achieve and therefore both cheaper and less likely to produce dose-dependent adverse events than further improvements. Trials have shown that it is worth, for example, forcing down blood pressure to the tightest limits in the highest-risk patients, but many will not tolerate the treatment. The large diabetes trials showed that tighter blood glucose control was beneficial, but was associated with more hypoglycaemic episodes. For this reason the outcomes shown in trials are often not achieved, and therefore presumably the full benefits on mortality and morbidity are not produced either.

The balance

A difficult balance may have to be set between achieving the desired outcome initially intended and forcing the patient to take so much medication that they suffer adverse events that affect compliance, and possibly even cause harm. This does not invalidate the concept of setting high goals to achieve; it merely means that monitoring for adverse events is as important as monitoring for the positive outcome desired. If a patient is seen as an individual, and their quality of life considered important, then the questions about risk and cost against any benefits will be easier to answer.

 ## PH3: The detailed assessment of each problem

This will consist of several thoughts:
- How serious or urgent is this problem?
- Is there a drug-related reason why the patient has this problem?

- Is the desired outcome being met? If not, why not?
- Is it being treated appropriately?
- Are there any exacerbating factors?
- What has been tried already? Did it help?

The detailed assessment of a patient's problems is carried out to help the healthcare professional to identify reasons for treatment failure (if any) and to decide what action needs to be taken for each problem.

First, any treatment that the patient is currently receiving for a particular problem needs to be identified. Relating the drug treatment being received to each problem in this manner is more likely to produce rational decisions than the reverse. The next step requires a consideration of what may have contributed to each problem or why the aims of treatment are not currently being met. Factors that may have contributed to the patient's problem can be divided into concurrent diseases (e.g. a patient admitted following a stroke who is hypertensive and diabetic) or medication being taken. Examples of the latter include patients with neutropenia who are taking clozapine, or patients with acute renal failure who are taking naproxen or angiotensin-converting enzyme inhibitors (ACEIs). In some cases there may be several possible factors contributing to the patient's problem.

In considering each pharmaceutical care problem, it may be useful to use a 'sieve' based on the 'drug-related problem' categories defined by Hepler and Strand[1] and subsequent work.[2,3]

Could the pharmaceutical care problem be caused, aggravated or insufficiently controlled by:
- **the patient suffering from an adverse event** (e.g. the patient is constipated while taking dihydrocodeine)?
- **the patient receiving drug therapy without a clear indication** (e.g. lansoprazole continued for years in an otherwise healthy patient)?
- **the patient not receiving a drug despite there being a clear indication** (e.g. with coronary heart disease but no statin)?
- **the patient receiving an inappropriate or less appropriate therapy** (e.g. bendroflumethiazide

to treat severe oedema when a loop diuretic is needed)?

- **the patient receiving too little or too much of a suitable therapy** (e.g. amitriptyline 10 mg to treat depression; initial dose of codeine 60 mg qds in a frail elderly patient)?
- **the patient not receiving or not taking a suitable therapy that has actually been prescribed** (e.g. patient has difficulty obtaining further supplies or is non-compliant)?

 ## PH4: Consideration of other problems and co-morbidity

Many of the patients whom pharmacists encounter will suffer from more than one medical condition and can be described as having co-morbidities. Patients may be at risk of developing diseases due to them suffering from another one, e.g. ischaemic heart disease in a hypertensive patient. With an increasingly elderly population, the existence of co-morbidities in patients is likely to become more prevalent in future years. The presence of co-morbidities can have a significant impact on the care of the patient.

Exacerbation of another problem

Inadequate control of one condition may adversely affect the control of another, e.g. a patient with ischaemic heart disease and iron deficiency anaemia who has a low haemoglobin is at risk of increased episodes of chest pain.

Increased significance of another problem

Hypertension and diabetes are both significant problems that a patient may have. However, coexistence of these two problems greatly increases the risk of renal disease, ischaemic heart disease and stroke.

Differential diagnoses

A patient's presenting symptoms may be attributable to more than one of their medical conditions, e.g. shortness of breath may be due to worsening heart failure or an acute exacerbation of chronic obstructive pulmonary disease (COPD), or the development of a new problem such as pulmonary embolism.

Drug choice

The presence of other co-morbidities can impact on the choice of drug prescribed for the patient:

- Coexistence of some diseases contraindicates the use of some drugs, e.g. metformin in renal failure, verapamil in heart failure, clopidogrel in active bleeding. In other cases the drug may not be contraindicated but cautioned, e.g. antidepressants in epilepsy (due to the risk of lowering the seizure threshold).
- Renal and hepatic impairment can affect the way the patient handles drugs and necessitate a reduction in dose or avoidance of a particular drug. Hepatic impairment does not usually affect drug handling significantly unless severe, whereas even mild renal impairment may require dose reduction or complete avoidance of certain drugs.

Pregnancy and breast feeding

These are factors that require consideration in a similar manner to co-morbidities when managing other medical conditions, and have a major impact on drug choice.

Polypharmacy

Co-morbidities are a major factor in patients receiving polypharmacy, which can create problems with patient compliance. In addition, polypharmacy increases the likelihood of patients experiencing drug interactions and adverse effects.

 ## PH5: Treatment options available and the preferred option

Once the problem has been properly assessed, either it will be:

- controlled (outcomes of care met) and not treated

- controlled (outcomes of care met) and being treated in some way
- uncontrolled (outcomes of care not met) and not treated
- uncontrolled (outcomes of care not met) and being treated in some way.

Controlled problems

Where the outcomes of care are being met without drug treatment, obviously the introduction of a drug therapy is not required. If a controlled problem is being treated with medication, even if the treatment may not fall neatly into the latest guidelines, it may be best left alone. The exceptions to this might include situations such as:

- other treatment choices that are known to offer additional benefits/better adverse event profiles than the current therapy
- other treatment choices that fit better with known co-morbidity (less likely to aggravate another problem/more likely to help it)
- the patient who is experiencing an adverse effect from the current therapy
- the current therapy that is probably unnecessary.

Uncontrolled problems

If a problem is currently uncontrolled, that is, the desired outcomes are not being achieved, then some action is needed. Drug therapy may need to be stopped, started or modified. The options for treating different conditions are increasingly evidence based and published by organisations such as NICE.

The National Institute for Health and Clinical Excellence

This is an NHS body intended to remove 'postcode prescribing' by promoting best practice based on clinical evidence. Some practitioners feel that its guidance is sometimes too restrictive but it should be remembered that it is defining the minimum level of care throughout the NHS. NICE guidance, or the lack of such, should not be used to withhold treatment required by patients, though there is a perception, at least in the popular press, that this can occur in practice.

Professional body statements

In this book we refer heavily to consensus statements from bodies such as the British Hypertension Society and British Thoracic Society (BTS). Their current recommendations may demand a tighter control of conditions than that required by NICE, or access to a wider range of drugs. This merely reflects a slightly different agenda in their preparation – with more medical and less political/financial input. In addition, evidence changes over time, and guidance often becomes out of date very quickly.

Local guidelines

Most NHS hospital and primary care trusts (PCTs) have local formularies to implement NICE and professional guidance, specifying a choice of drug as well as a preferred class. These guidelines are usually binding on practitioners working in those organisations, at least for initial management choices.

Cost–benefit

If one option is much more cost-effective than another, then it is in the public interest to use it in preference to more expensive therapies. This decision may already have been taken into account in the guidelines referred to above. The more expensive therapy may well remain available for those who fail to tolerate or do not achieve their desired outcome on the standard therapy. Acquisition cost alone may be too narrow a consideration – the likelihood of achieving an outcome, safety profile and monitoring costs needs to be considered.

Risk management

Where two drugs have differing adverse effect rates or profiles, this needs to be factored into the consideration as to the preferred therapy. Risk management may dictate the use of heparin in prefilled syringes, for example, even though this adds to the acquisition cost.

Licence

If one treatment possibility is licensed for the use for which it is intended, it is usually the treatment of choice over an unlicensed therapy in initial use.

Ease of monitoring

Whether a drug needs complex monitoring may affect its selection. Many hospitals have switched to using expensive subcutaneous low-molecular-weight heparins (LMWHs) rather than infusions of unfractionated heparin to treat thromboembolism. In addition to any clinical benefits, the increased acquisition cost of the drug is offset by the removal of the need to send samples of blood to the haematology laboratory or to buy infusion pumps. In addition, the removal of the need to monitor, which may get forgotten in practice, removes the danger of under- or over-treatment of a serious condition. Finally, there is a major saving in staff time, especially nursing time, which is both a cost saving and a quality gain.

Co-morbidity

This has been discussed in the previous section, but clearly co-morbidity is an important consideration in drug use. It may create compelling indications for, or contraindications to, the use of a particular therapy.

Past experience and patient preferences

The assessment will have generated information on what has been tried for a particular problem. Has it worked? Was it tolerated?

The preferred choice of action

Having considered where the patient is at in relation to any current guidelines, and the additional factors above, the next step to be advocated may become clear. You may have decided to advocate no change at all or you may desire to recommend:
- a dose change
- an additional drug
- a different drug, formulation or route of administration
- a cessation of therapy.

Now you need to ensure implementation of your advice.

 PH6: Implementation: whether, when and how to act

Having identified the problem, considered the outcome to be achieved and the possible routes to that goal in terms of different therapeutic options, pharmaceutical care involves implementation of your chosen solution if it is not to become simply a philosophical exercise. Once the preferred option becomes clear, implementation involves three overlapping elements (Figure 1.6).

Whether to act

As Kenny Rogers sang in 'The Gambler' in 1978, 'You got to know when to hold 'em, know when to fold 'em; know when to walk away'. In any decision, three possibilities open up (Figure 1.7).

Whether to act: how to decide

In many situations, the need to act will be self-evident, or the organisation for which you work

Figure 1.6 Elements of implementation

```
                    WHETHER TO ACT

              PREFERRED THERAPEUTIC
                     ACTION

WHEN TO ACT   ◄──────────►      HOW TO ACT
```

Figure 1.7 Possibilities in making a decision

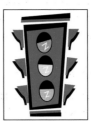

RED: DO NOTHING
Based on the classic adage, 'If it ain't broke, then don't fix it' often no action is necessary, other than making a commitment to review the patient again at a suitable interval.

AMBER: WAIT
The problem seems not quite controlled or prevented, or it is still unstable. However, immediate action may not be necessary. Examples might include:
• awaiting a recheck of serum electrolytes
• seeing if a patient becomes more proficient in using an inhaler device
• giving epoetin time to achieve its expected effect.
*Any action that involves waiting must contain some assurance that the required review **will** take place, even if the patient moves beyond your care.*

GREEN: ACT NOW
Pharmacists, if accepting their professional responsibilities, need to be suggesting the initiation of a drug, the change of a drug or dose, or the cessation of a particular therapy. (Of course, supplementary and independent prescribers may act themselves in certain circumstances.) If the prescriber declines this advice, the pharmacist needs to make a further decision whether to accept this or not.

Figure 1.8 How to decide whether to act

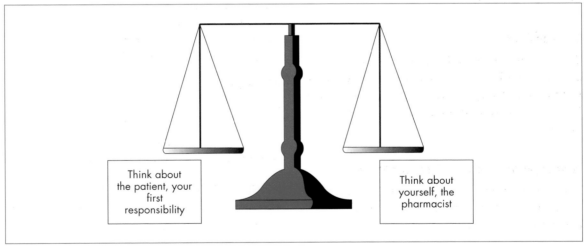

Think about the patient, your first responsibility

Think about yourself, the pharmacist

may have guidelines on required responses to take in specific circumstances, for example, where a dose is seemingly excessive. But in other situations, pharmacists will need to use some judgement as to whether to act or not – inexperienced pharmacists often use one of two models to assist them in that decision (Figure 1.8). Both, surprisingly, can be effective.

These approaches can be summed up as one of two thoughts:

1. 'If it were my grandmother (or brother/sister etc.)' – considering the **consequences to the patient,** an approach that asks: 'What is in the patient's best interest and what would I want done if he or she were a relative of mine?'

2. 'Cover your back' – a more selfishly defensive approach that considers the **consequences to the pharmacist**: 'What is the worst thing that might happen if I fail to act, and what risks am I creating by suggesting this change?' A pharmacist should never walk away from a patient if their self-protection instinct for their own reputation and career is telling them they should be doing more. Junior pharmacists may also wish to involve more experienced colleagues in assisting with this decision.

'BRAN' Some healthcare professionals like to use approaches such as the acronym BRAN to assist decision making, once their possible action has suggested itself:

Benefits?   What are these for the patient?
Risks?   What are these for the patient?
Action?   What might happen if I act?
No action?   What might happen if I do not act?

Examples of situations where most pharmacists would consider failure to act as negligent

- The initiation of a prescription for diltiazem in a patient with symptomatic heart failure
- The pharmacist is aware of an important medication that the patient takes regularly at home which has not been continued on admission, without documentation in the notes or obvious cause, or which has been omitted at discharge from hospital (note: they should always ask themselves 'Why might it have been discontinued?' before intervening)
- The addition of an interacting drug such as amiodarone to a prescription for regular warfarin, when the patient is not under frequent supervision
- The prescription of a month's supply of high-dose steroids where the existence of a long-term inflammatory condition is not known to the pharmacist or patient
- The prescription of a drug well outside its *British National Formulary* (*BNF*) dose, or in a contraindicated or cautioned condition, without the reason known to the pharmacist.

Examples of situations where small delay may well be acceptable or even preferable

- A patient has been taking steroids for several years; should bisphosphonates be prescribed?
- A patient has been taking simvastatin for two years without having their lipids measured; should this help?
- A renal patient on Epoetin has a haemoglobin of 9 g/dL – do they need iron studies with a view to prescribing iron or an increased dose of Epoetin?
- A patient on ferrous sulphate in the long term, but who has a lot of nausea and is willing to try an alternative formulation.

When to act

> ACT IMMEDIATELY IF THE FAILURE TO ACT MIGHT RESULT IN HARM.

However, apart from the situations referred to previously where further information is being awaited, not all interventions need to be made immediately. Some will require action by immediately contacting a doctor or amending a prescription, and others can be deferred to a ward round, or by raising the issue with a doctor at a more convenient time. Hospital pharmacists quickly learn not to bleep doctors to discuss issues that can wait, unless the patient is being discharged immediately. They may be attending ward rounds, having a break or talking to patients or relatives. In primary care, scheduled feedback times can be agreed, rather than interrupting busy surgery sessions. A friendly and productive relationship with the medical and nursing staff is maintained by some consideration of the pressures on other professional groups.

How to act

If, as Hepler and Strand argued, the ultimate aim of pharmaceutical care is to improve the patient's quality of life,[1] then all the pharmaceutical care planning in the world will not improve the patient's lot if the doctor cannot be convinced to act on your advice.

How to act: factors that assist the intervention

Relationship with prescribers. Pharmaceutical care requires a relationship between the prescriber and the pharmacist. The better the relationship, the greater the contribution to pharmaceutical care as more interventions will be voiced. Where the doctor and pharmacist are not well known to each other, for example:

- a pharmacist based in the hospital dispensary while checking discharge prescriptions
- a community pharmacist dealing with GP-generated prescriptions),

the relationship might consist only of the briefest of introductions and courtesies, and only the most pressing interventions may be made, such as those listed on p. 18 as demanding immediate action.

Where the relationship between the prescriber and pharmacist is established and functional, for example:

- a junior pharmacist visiting a hospital ward every day and chatting to the junior medical staff
- a pharmacist regularly joining the consultant or registrar ward round
- a primary care pharmacist contracted to the GP to provide medication review,

then the less urgent, but no less important, interventions may be made effectively.

Pharmacists and pharmacy departments should use every opportunity to build good relationships with the prescribers with whom they work. So, in hospitals, greet them each time you pass on wards, follow up queries thoroughly, ensure that they have had their *BNF* and local information. Pharmacists should be involved in ward rounds, discharge planning, medical staff induction and social activities. Calls to all areas of the pharmacy department should be answered politely and effectively, and pharmacists should develop links such as participation in education, induction and policy formation wherever possible. A poor reputation for your profession will be engendered by departments for which the most frequent contact with junior doctors is to demand their presence to correct controlled drug prescriptions. Similar opportunities will exist in primary care.

Involving others. If the query is not urgent, it may be much more effective to pass the query on to a pharmacist with a closer involvement with the team. Even if the query is urgent and you are unable to generate action, most pharmacists and technicians work with more senior colleagues to whom the problem can be handed over.

Time. If the patient is not going to move beyond your care, waiting while more information is gathered or a better time to intervene with the prescriber presents itself, as discussed above, may enable a more effective intervention to be made. Most people prefer to be presented with solutions, not merely problems, and prescribers are no different.

Courtesy and confidence. These are the results of a good relationship with the prescriber. But even if that relationship is unformed at the time of intervention, anyone can *be* courteous just as anyone can *appear* confident. Armed with these two weapons, your successful intervention rate will rise. It is important to remember that confidence in your intervention is not the same as dogmatic belief. Overconfidence can be dangerous, such as when junior doctors are persuaded to represcribe aspirin missing on a newly admitted patient's prescription, without considering whether there was a reason for this omission. For many interventions, even experienced pharmacists will simply lay their concern before a senior medical staff member in a concise and confident manner, and then let them decide whether the action is appropriate.

Liability. Doctors are well aware that, if a pharmacist suggests an intervention designed to prevent harm or close a serious omission, and they fail to act, then they will be liable in law. (They are also aware that you may well have documented the interaction.) Of course, this liability risk works against you when you are trying to make an intervention that is less urgent, and they are aware that taking action may create risks whilst inaction may seem safer. Sometimes junior hospital doctors may be unwilling to change prescriptions because they are anxious about getting it wrong or facing the disapproval of their seniors. It may be appropriate to allow them to raise the issue with more experienced medical staff on an imminent ward round – it all depends on the circumstances.

Inexperience. Junior pharmacists and preregistration graduates often feel inadequate after making harsh comparisons between their performance and that of more senior colleagues. However, your inexperience can be a powerful weapon in helping the patient. For example, on hospital ward rounds, even junior pharmacists can say things such as, 'I haven't done much rheumatology but I was wondering if . . .', or 'I have read the NICE guidance, but I would be glad to know your policy on starting statins after myocardial infarction in heart failure'. Most consultants will respond very positively to the chance to share their knowledge.

Implementation: patient opinion

It is important to consider the opinions of the patient on any proposed changes to their therapy. In primary care, they may have had a relationship with their GP built up over many years. The building of trust and the securing of concordance is as important between pharmacists and technicians and patients as it is between patients and their doctors. What will the patient think of your intervention? Even if you don't think their antihypertensive is still the most evidence-based choice, will they feel railroaded if it is changed? Will they take

it? Will they see it as a cost-saving measure? What if their new treatment causes adverse events?

Implementation: final thoughts

In the absence of a standard description of pharmaceutical care or consistent levels of staffing in the NHS, different hospitals and primary care organisations will adopt different levels of depth of care provision. You have to live with this and adopt the highest level of practice that your situation allows. However, in no situation should pharmacists be providing care that does not even pass the hurdle required to avoid an allegation of negligence. It is not always appropriate to make every intervention theoretically possible. Medicines carry risks even when prescribed appropriately, and patients respond in complex and idiosyncratic ways to changes in therapy. As said earlier, 'If it ain't broke, don't fix it'.

At the end of the day, unless you are a supplementary prescriber pharmacist acting within a defined clinical management plan, it is the prescriber who has the ultimate responsibility for prescribing and the bulk of the legal liability. Except in the most urgent and important of interventions, some recognition of this is important in your interaction.

PH7: Monitoring: for effect and for adverse effects

Hepler and Strand observed that failure to monitor patients' drug therapy was the most important omission made by healthcare professionals.[1] All patients receiving drug therapy require some degree of monitoring. Monitoring is required for two reasons (Figure 1.9).

Figure 1.9 Purposes of monitoring

To ensure the efficacy of drug therapy

To ensure the safety of drug therapy

Efficacy and adverse effects

Reference to the initial desired outcomes of therapy will ensure that these have been achieved. For example, if the desired outcome of therapy was to reduce blood pressure to below 140/80 mmHg, then monitoring will check whether this has been achieved. If it has not been, then reassessment of the patient will be necessary and further interventions suggested until the goal has been met. In a similar manner, monitoring will ensure that the desired outcome of therapy has been achieved without aggravating or creating other problems. For example, the use of beta-blockers to achieve the blood pressure reduction above may have led to cold extremities, tiredness, breathlessness or other problems.

What to monitor

Monitoring can be qualitative (e.g. patients' reported pain) or quantitative (e.g. blood glucose). Monitoring parameters include blood tests, physical measurements (e.g. pulse, blood pressure) or simply talking to patients to assess their response to drug therapy (e.g. frequency of angina attacks, pain control). Some monitoring parameters are carried out to ensure both the safety and efficacy of drug therapy, e.g. a patient commenced on an ACEI for hypertension should have their blood pressure monitored to ensure that the target blood pressure is being achieved but not excessively exceeded to a dangerous degree.

Once the monitoring parameters for each problem have been identified, a decision has to be made regarding the frequency of monitoring, to ensure that problems with drug therapy are identified at an early stage without inconveniencing the patient. For example, clozapine therapy initially requires weekly full blood counts to identify the development of any dyscrasias. If this recommendation is not adhered to the patient could develop unnoticed neutropenia and sepsis from opportunistic infections, which could have been prevented if low neutrophils had been identified earlier. Conversely, there is little point checking a patient's haemoglobin weekly to identify whether oral iron therapy is having the desired effect.

A consideration of time to response and the drug's half-life therefore help to determine the frequency of monitoring that each problem requires and the likely time to presentation of adverse drug reactions. For example, pulmonary fibrosis with methotrexate or osteoporosis with oral steroids is likely to present later than acute renal failure after an ACEI is initiated.

Finally, monitoring the patient's perception of their therapy is vital to promote compliance and ensure concordance. It has been said that the most expensive drug therapy is that which the patient will not take.

Summary: adopting a holistic approach

Reassembling the case

A patient is more than a set of different problems. Depending on local policy, a pharmaceutical care plan needs to be drawn up either in the pharmacist's mind or, more appropriately, on paper or electronically. This need not be complicated, and one helpful factor is that the order of priority of interventions for implementation is usually (but not always) in the same order of prioritisation as the original problem list.

For each problem, after assessment and consideration of the therapeutic options, there may be one or more desired changes to implement, as discussed in the chapters on **implementation PH6** and associated **monitoring** (**PH7**). If a documentary system is adopted, these can be listed alongside each of the prioritised problems. This is your pharmaceutical care plan (Table 1.4). Practical examples of care planning are found in Section 3.

Reassessing the patient

In addition to the cyclical nature of the handling of each individual problem, there should also be, at appropriate intervals, a re-evaluation of the whole patient. These intervals depend very much on the condition of the patient and might be daily following an acute hospital admission, or annually in the case of a patient with no changing or acute needs in primary care. At re-evaluation, problems may:

- have changed priority (e.g. blood pressure well controlled but lipids now high)
- have resolved to the point that they may be excluded from further consideration (e.g. chest infection resolved)
- have developed that were not present at the original assessment and need outcomes defining and assessment (e.g. the patient is found to have type 2 diabetes mellitus).

Table 1.4

Pharmaceutical care plan for .... DOB .... Allergies				
Problem (prioritised for action)	Desired outcome(s) of treatment	Detailed assessment: Current therapy? Controlled or not? Severity? Causes? Previous therapy?	Treatment options and implementation	Monitoring
1				
2				
3				
4				
5				

Chart 1.1 The pharmaceutical care cycle

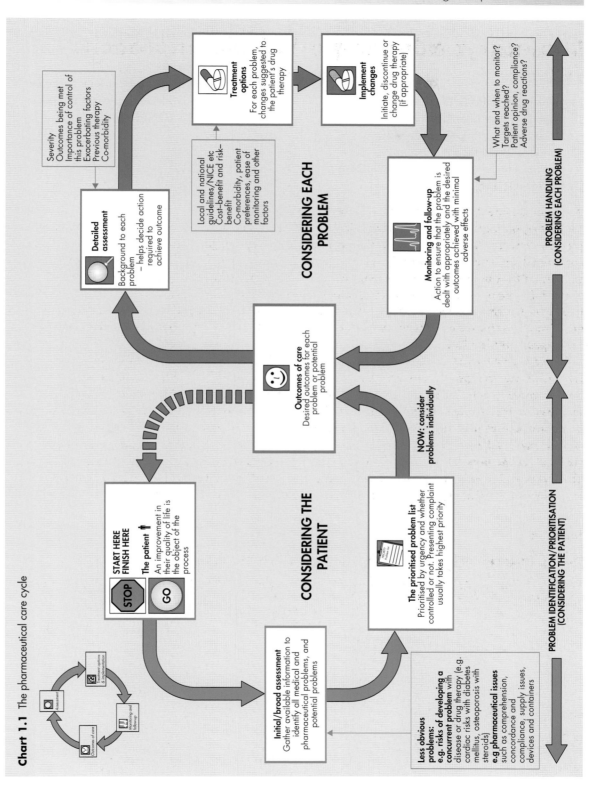

Detailed assessment
Background to each problem
– helps decide action required to achieve outcome

Severity
Outcomes being met
Importance of control of this problem
Exacerbating factors
Previous therapy
Co-morbidity

Treatment options
For each problem, changes suggested to the patient's drug therapy

Local and national guidelines/NICE etc
Cost–benefit and risk–benefit
Co-morbidity, patient preferences, ease of monitoring and other factors

Implement changes
Initiate, discontinue or change drug therapy (if appropriate)

CONSIDERING EACH PROBLEM

Monitoring and follow-up
Action to ensure that the problem is dealt with appropriately and the desired outcomes achieved with minimal adverse effects

What and when to monitor?
Targets reached?
Patient opinion, compliance?
Adverse drug reactions?

PROBLEM HANDLING
(CONSIDERING EACH PROBLEM)

Outcomes of care
Desired outcomes for each problem or potential problem

NOW: consider problems individually

START HERE
FINISH HERE

The patient
An improvement in their quality of life is the object of the process

STOP

GO

CONSIDERING THE PATIENT

The prioritised problem list
Prioritised by urgency and whether controlled or not. Presenting complaint usually takes highest priority

Initial/broad assessment
Gather available information to identify all medical and pharmaceutical problems, and potential problems

Less obvious problems:
e.g. risks of developing a concurrent problem with disease or drug therapy (e.g. cardiac risks with diabetes mellitus, osteoporosis with steroids)
e.g pharmaceutical issues such as comprehension, concordance and compliance, supply issues, devices and containers

PROBLEM IDENTIFICATION/PRIORITISATION
(CONSIDERING THE PATIENT)

The cyclical flow of the pharmaceutical care process is shown in Chart 1.1.

References

1 Hepler C, Strand L. Opportunities and responsibilities in pharmaceutical care. *Am J Hosp Pharm* 1990; 47: 533–543.

2 Strand L. Building a practice in pharmaceutical care. *Pharm J* 1998; 260: 87–86. (ONLINE)

3 Cippole RJ, Strand L, Morley PC. *Pharmaceutical Care Practice*. New York: McGraw-Hill; 1998.

4 Simpson D. What is medicines management and what is pharmaceutical care? *Pharm J* 2001; 266: 150. (ONLINE)

Section 2

The Problems

Many chronic conditions have established pathways of care and preferred first choices of therapy established, hopefully, from large-scale clinical trials. These pathways are increasingly internationalised as the evidence base from which they are established is available globally. Of course, it is the patient being treated, not the pathway, and therapy is individualised in the light of the assessment and local policy. This choice then needs to be implemented, and since few pharmacists are currently prescribers this will involve achieving co-operation of medical staff. Finally, and most importantly, the effects of therapy need to be monitored. Have the desired outcomes of therapy been achieved, and has the patient suffered adverse events that are diminishing quality of life?

These guidelines are not the only ones available for different conditions, and new consensus guidelines, policy from government bodies and opinion are emerging constantly. It is the responsibility of the pharmacist to keep up to date with best practice.

It is important to remember that patients are individuals, and all choices should be made with that view in mind. Guidelines are meant to inform, not dictate, prescribing recommendations.

C Cardiology

Chapter contents

The assistance of Catherine Lee, MRPharmS, Senior Cardiology Pharmacist at the Royal Liverpool University Hospital, is gratefully acknowledged in the preparation of this section.

Introduction

The majority of patients admitted to medical wards in a hospital, or reviewed in primary care due to multiple drug therapy, will have a cardiac problem. The four most common conditions encountered are listed below.

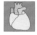 ### Problem 1: the patient has chronic hypertension

This condition is both common and commonly undiagnosed. Untreated, it is associated with an increased morbidity and mortality from cardiovascular disease (CVD). Diabetes makes hypertension particularly dangerous, and both diabetes and hypertension are becoming more common as the population grows more obese and less active, and contains a growing number of people from ethnic minorities and older age groups.

 ### Problem 2: the patient has ischaemic heart disease

Ischaemic heart disease, often caused by hypertension, diabetes and dyslipidaemia, results in narrowing of the coronary arteries and pain (angina) because of a failure to meet myocardial oxygen demand. The more common manifestation, known as stable angina, is discussed here and should not be confused with unstable angina, part of the acute coronary syndromes (ACSs). This does not mean that stable angina is always well controlled, or 'stable', however.

 ### Problem 3: the patient has heart failure

Hypertension, ischaemia, ventricular hypertrophy, myocardial infarction and other conditions can lead to heart failure, where the heart cannot meet the demand of the body for oxygen. The failure of the heart as a pump may lead to fluid accumulation in the lungs or lower limbs, or the patient may not yet be symptomatic, and the condition is associated with a high mortality. The condition is often undertreated, and yet therapies exist that have been proven to have substantial benefits.

 ### Problem 4: the patient needs to reduce their cardiovascular risk

Many seemingly healthy adults, as well as patients with the above conditions, are at a high risk of premature mortality. There are a number of strategies that are effective in reducing these risks at a population level.

The pharmacist's role

Many patients have co-morbidity – they have more than one type of cardiac condition or other medical conditions that will affect drug choice. In addition, they may end up on a multitude of different treatments, creating problems with interactions, adverse events and comprehension. Many treatments will not make the patient feel better; indeed they may make the patient feel worse, but are backed by evidence from large-scale trials of benefits in terms of reduced morbidity and mortality. Poor comprehension and concordance lead to poor compliance, and there are many opportunities for the pharmacist to intervene to optimise outcomes of therapy.

Cardiology 1 problem: the patient has chronic hypertension

 Objectives of this section

The reader should be able to detail:
- the objectives of care in hypertension
- the use of evidence-based guidelines to derive thresholds (when to initiate) and targets (desired quantitative result) of treatment
- the importance of non-drug measures and the promotion of compliance in achieving blood pressure (BP) reduction targets
- the importance of managing BP as part of overall CVD risk
- the main treatment options available:
  — beta-blockers
  — rate-limiting and non-rate-limiting calcium-channel blockers
  — thiazide diuretics
  — ACEIs and angiotensin II receptor antagonists
- monitoring required to ensure safety and efficacy of drug therapy.

 Further reading: basics

- *British National Formulary*, current edn. London: Royal Pharmaceutical Society and British Medical Association. Section 2.5: Drugs affecting the renin–angiotensin system and some other antihypertensive drugs. (ONLINE)
- Randall MD, Neil KE. *Disease Management*. London: Pharmaceutical Press; 2004. Chapter 11: Hypertension.

 Further reading: moving on

- Walker R, Edwards C, eds. *Clinical Pharmacy and Therapeutics*, 3rd edn. London: Churchill Livingstone; 2003. Chapter 17: Hypertension.
- Dodds LJ, ed. *Drugs in Use*, 3rd edn. London: Pharmaceutical Press; 2003. Chapter 3: Hypertension.

 Guidelines

- Williams B, Poulter NR, Brown MJ *et al*. British Hypertension Society guidelines for hypertension management 2004 (BHS-IV): summary. *BMJ* 2004; 328: 634–640. (ONLINE)
- National Institute for Clinical Excellence. *Clinical Guideline 34: Management of Hypertension in Adults in Primary Care*. London: NICE; 2006. (ONLINE)
- Department of Health. *National Service Framework for Coronary Heart Disease*. London: Department of Health; 2000. (ONLINE)

SAQ **Self-assessment questions: Cardiology 1** (Answers on p. 35)

1. What are the consequences of prolonged elevation in blood pressure?
2. Why is it important to maintain blood pressure within limits, even though these limits are constantly being revised?

(Questions continued on page 29)

Chart 2.1 Cardiology 1 problem: the patient has chronic hypertension

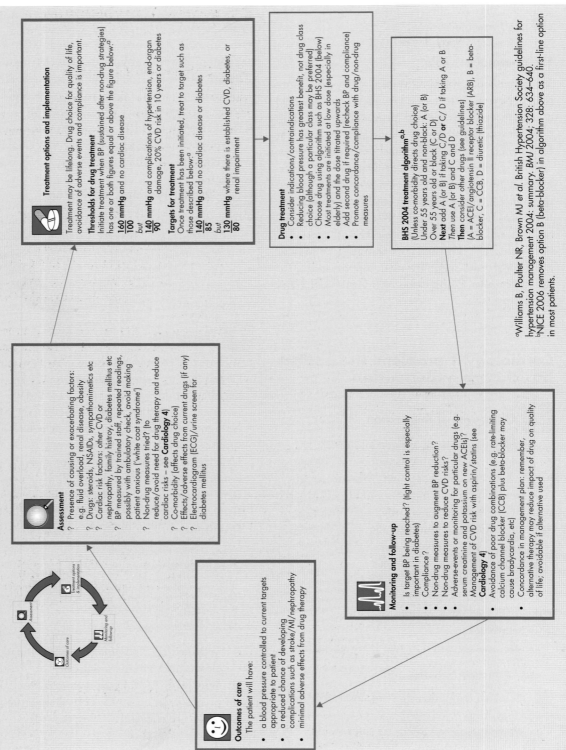

Assessment

? Presence of causing or exacerbating factors: e.g. fluid overload, renal disease, obesity
? Drugs: steroids, NSAIDs, sympathomimetics etc
? Cardiac risk factors: other CVD or nephropathy, family history, diabetes mellitus etc
? BP measured by trained staff, repeated readings, possibly with ambulatory check, avoid making patient anxious ('white coat syndrome')
? Non-drug measures tried? (to reduce/avoid need for drug therapy and reduce cardiac risks – see **Cardiology 4**)
? Co-morbidity (affects drug choice)
? Effects/adverse effects from current drugs (if any)
? Electrocardiogram (ECG)/urine screen for diabetes mellitus

Treatment options and implementation

Treatment may be lifelong. Drug choice for quality of life, avoidance of adverse events and compliance is important.

Thresholds for drug treatment

Initiate treatment when BP (sustained after non-drug strategies) has one or both figures equal or above the figure below:[a]

160 mmHg and no cardiac disease
100
but
140 mmHg and complications of hypertension, end-organ
90 damage, 20% CVD risk in 10 years or diabetes

Targets for treatment

Once treatment has been initiated, treat to target such as those described below:[a]

140 mmHg and no cardiac disease or diabetes
85
but
130 mmHg where there is established CVD, diabetes, or
80 renal impairment

Drug treatment

- Consider indications/contraindications
- Reducing blood pressure has greatest benefit, not drug class choice (although a particular class may be preferred
- Choose drug using algorithm such as BHS 2004 (below)
- Most treatments are initiated at low dose (especially in elderly) and the dose titrated upwards
- Add second drug if required (recheck BP and compliance)
- Promote concordance/compliance with drug/non-drug measures

BHS 2004 treatment algorithm[a,b]

(Unless co-morbidity directs drug choice)
Under 55 years old and non-black: A (or B)
Over 55 years old or black (C or D)
Next add A (or B) if taking C/D **or** C/D if taking A or B
Then use A (or B) and C and D
Then consider other drugs (see guidelines)
(A = ACEI/angiotensin II receptor blocker (ARB), B = beta-blocker, C = CCB, D = diuretic (thiazide)

[a]Williams B, Poulter NR, Brown MJ *et al.* British Hypertension Society guidelines for hypertension management 2004: summary. *BMJ* 2004; 328: 634–640.
[b]NICE 2006 removes option B (beta-blocker) in algorithm above as a first-line option in most patients.

Monitoring and follow-up

- Is target BP being reached? (tight control is especially important in diabetes)
- Compliance?
- Non-drug measures to augment BP reduction?
- Non-drug measures to reduce CVD risks?
- Adverse-events or monitoring for particular drugs (e.g. serum creatinine and potassium on new ACEIs)
- Management of CVD risk with aspirin/statins (see **Cardiology 4**)
- Avoidance of poor drug combinations (e.g. rate-limiting calcium channel blocker (CCB) plus beta-blocker may cause bradycardia, etc)
- Concordance in management plan: remember, alternative therapy may reduce impact of drug on quality of life; avoidable if alternative used

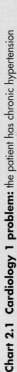

Outcomes of care

The patient will have:

- a blood pressure controlled to current targets appropriate to patient
- a reduced chance of developing complications such as stroke/MI/nephropathy
- minimal adverse effects from drug therapy

SAQ Self-assessment questions:
Cardiology 1 (continued)

3. What is the difference between a target and a threshold in the management of hypertension?

4. Is there such a thing as a blood pressure that is too low?

5. Why are people with established cardio-vascular disease, diabetes, or kidney damage treated at lower thresholds and to tighter targets than the rest of the population?

6. Should non-drug measures always be tried before initiating drug therapy?

7. How should drug therapy be initiated?

8. Why is the consideration of additional measures to reduce cardiovascular risk important?

9. Which is the best drug with which to start treatment?

10. Table 2.1 offers some simple guidance as to the appropriateness of drug selection for hypertension in different types of patient. How does co-morbidity affect drug choice by the prescriber or pharmacist?

Cardiology 2 problem: the patient has ischaemic heart disease

 Objectives of this section

The reader should be able to detail:

- the objectives of care in ischaemic heart disease
- the importance of controlling exacerbating factors and co-morbidity
- The treatment options available:
  — aspirin
  — beta-blockers
  — rate-limiting calcium-channel blockers (RLCCBs)
  — non-rate-limiting 'dihydropyridine' calcium-channel blockers (DHP-CCBs)
  — nitrates, for 'when required use' and prophylactic use (usually sustained release)
  — nicorandil
- lifestyle changes and drug therapy to reduce symptoms and reduce risk of cardiovascular death (dealt with more fully in **Cardiology 4**)
- monitoring required to ensure efficacy and safety of drug therapy.

Table 2.1 Co-morbidity and drug choice in hypertension: some examples

Drug class	Good choice	Poor choice
ACEIs/ARBs (in general ARBs are preferred if patient has cough or other non-shared adverse drug reaction (ADR) on ACEI therapy)	Heart failure; diabetic nephropathy left ventricular dysfunction after myocardial infarction (MI) or left ventricular hypertrophy	Pregnancy; renovascular disease (stenosis). Careful monitoring needed in renal impairment to detect any deterioration
Beta-blockers	MI/symptomatic ischaemic heart disease (IHD) (angina)	Asthma/COPD; bradycardia; heart failure (except special use – see **Cardiology 3**). See NICE Guidance 2006 for further comment on beta-blocker use in hypertension
Calcium-channel blockers – dihydropyridines (DHP-CCBs)	Older patients; isolated systolic hypertension. Angina where rate-limiting CCBs not suitable (e.g. in heart failure)	
Rate-limiting calcium-channel blockers (RLCCBs)	Angina; older patients	Heart failure, with beta-blockers
Thiazides (diuretics)	Older patients; isolated systolic hypertension	Care in gout

Chart 2.2 Cardiology 2 problem: the patient has ischaemic heart disease

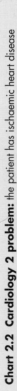

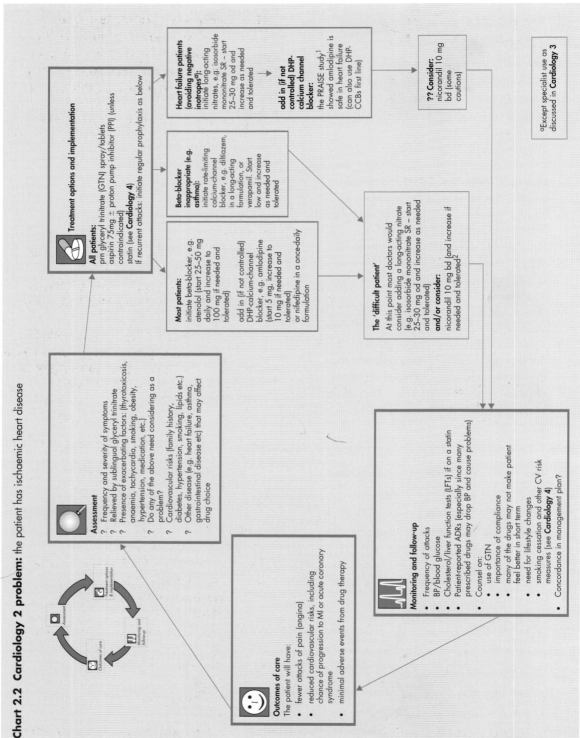

Assessment

? Frequency and severity of symptoms
? Relieved by sublingual glyceryl trinitrate
? Presence of exacerbating factors: (thyrotoxicosis, anaemia, tachycardia, smoking, obesity, hypertension, medication, etc.)
? Do any of the above need considering as a problem?
? Cardiovascular risks (family history, diabetes, hypertension, smoking, lipids etc.)
? Other disease (e.g. heart failure, asthma, gastrointestinal disease etc) that may affect drug choice

Outcomes of care

The patient will have:

• fewer attacks of pain (angina)
• reduced cardiovascular risks, including chance of progression to MI or acute coronary syndrome
• minimal adverse events from drug therapy

Monitoring and follow-up

• Frequency of attacks
• BP/blood glucose
• Cholesterol/liver function tests (LFTs) if on a statin
• Patient-reported ADRs (especially since many prescribed drugs may drop BP and cause problems)
• Counsel on:
  • use of GTN
  • importance of compliance
  • many of the drugs may not make patient feel better in short term
  • need for lifestyle changes
  • smoking cessation and other CV risk measures (see **Cardiology 4**)
• Concordance in management plan?

Treatment options and implementation

All patients:
prn glyceryl trinitrate (GTN) spray/tablets
aspirin 75mg ± proton pump inhibitor (PPI) (unless contraindicated)
statin (see **Cardiology 4**)
If recurrent attacks: initiate regular prophylaxis as below

Most patients:
initiate beta-blocker, e.g. atenolol (start 25–50 mg daily and increase to 100 mg if needed and tolerated)

add in (if not controlled) DHP-calcium-channel blocker, e.g. amlodipine (start 5 mg, increase to 10 mg if needed and tolerated) or nifedipine in a once-daily formulation

Beta-blocker inappropriate (e.g. asthma):
initiate rate-limiting calcium-channel blocker, e.g. diltiazem, in a long-acting formulation, or verapamil. Start low and increase as needed and tolerated

Heart failure patients (avoiding negative inotropes[a]):
initiate long-acting nitrates, e.g. isosorbide mononitrate SR – start 25–30 mg od and increase as needed and tolerated

add in (if not controlled) DHP-calcium channel blocker:
the PRAISE study[1] showed amlodipine is safe in heart failure (can also use DHP-CCBs first line)

The 'difficult patient'
At this point most doctors would consider adding a long-acting nitrate (e.g. isosorbide mononitrate SR – start 25–30 mg od and increase as needed and tolerated)
and/or consider:
nicorandil 10 mg bd (and increase if needed and tolerated[2]

?? Consider:
nicorandil 10 mg bd (some cautions)

[a]Except specialist use as discussed in **Cardiology 3**

Further reading: basics

- Randall MD, Neil KE (2003). *Disease Management*. London: Pharmaceutical Press; 2003. Chapter 13: Ischaemic heart disease.
- *British National Formulary*, current edn. London: Royal Pharmaceutical Society and British Medical Association. Section 2.5: Angina. (ONLINE)

 Further reading: moving on

- Williams H, Stevens M. Heart disease (2) chronic stable angina. *Pharm J* 2002; 269: 363–365. (ONLINE)
- Department of Health. *National Service Framework for Coronary Heart Disease*. London: Department of Health; 2000. (ONLINE)
- Walker R, Edwards C, eds. *Clinical Pharmacy and Therapeutics*, 3rd edn. London: Churchill-Livingstone; 2003. Chapter 18: Coronary heart disease.
- Dodds LJ, ed. *Drugs in Use*, 3rd edn. London: Pharmaceutical Press; 2003. Chapter 2: Ischaemic heart disease.

SAQ Self-assessment questions: **Cardiology 2** (Answers on p. 38)

1. What counselling is required when supplying a patient with glyceryl trinitrate (GTN) tablets for sublingual use?
2. What advantages and disadvantages does GTN spray offer over sublingual tablet formulations?
3. If a patient fails to tolerate aspirin 75 mg daily, should clopidogrel be used instead?
4. A patient is taking aspirin and atenolol 100 mg daily to control their angina, but is still getting attacks. What would the next approach be?
5. What is the place of dihydropyridine calcium-channel blockers in therapy?

6. Should diabetic patients, and those suffering from peripheral vascular disease, chronic obstructive pulmonary disease (COPD) or asthma avoid beta-blockers?
7. What is the role of nicorandil in angina therapy?
8. Should angina patients receive a statin therapy?

References

1 Packer M, O'Connor CM, Ghali JK, *et al.* Effect of amlodipine on morbidity and mortality in severe chronic heart failure (PRAISE Study). *N Engl J Med* 1996; 335: 1107–1114.
2 Iona Study Group. Effect of nicorandil on coronary events in patients with stable angina: the Impact Of Nicorandil in Angina (IONA) randomised trial. *Lancet* 2002; 359: 1269–1275.

Cardiology 3 problem: the patient has chronic heart failure

 Objectives of this section

The reader should be able to detail:
- the objectives of care in heart failure
- the importance of controlling exacerbating factors and co-morbidity
- the treatment options available:
  — loop diuretics
  — ACEIs and angiotensin II receptor blockers (ARBs)
  — beta-blockers
  — spironolactone
  — hydralazine/nitrates
  — digoxin
- monitoring required to ensure efficacy and safety of drug therapy.

Chart 2.3 Cardiology 3 problem: the patient has chronic heart failure

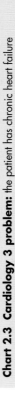

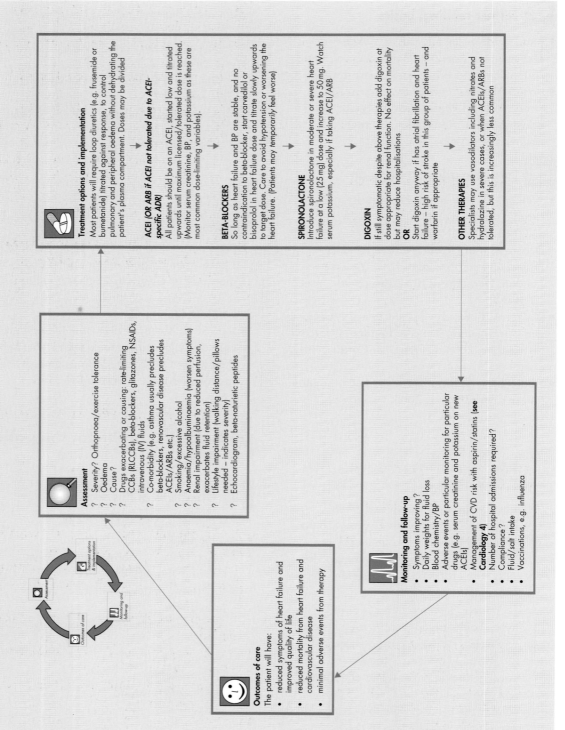

Assessment

- ? Severity? Orthopnoea/exercise tolerance
- ? Oedema
- ? Cause?
- ? Drugs exacerbating or causing: rate-limiting CCBs (RLCCBs), beta-blockers, glitazones, NSAIDs, intravenous (IV) fluids
- ? Co-morbidity (e.g. asthma usually precludes beta-blockers, renovascular disease precludes ACEIs/ARBs etc.)
- ? Smoking/excessive alcohol
- ? Anaemia/hypoalbuminaemia (worsen symptoms)
- ? Renal impairment (due to reduced perfusion, exacerbates fluid retention)
- ? Lifestyle impairment (walking distance/pillows needed – indicates severity)
- ? Echocardiogram, beta-natriuretic peptides

Outcomes of care

The patient will have:
- reduced symptoms of heart failure and improved quality of life
- reduced mortality from heart failure and cardiovascular disease
- minimal adverse events from therapy

Monitoring and follow-up

- Symptoms improving?
- Daily weights for fluid loss
- Blood chemistry/BP
- Adverse events or particular monitoring for particular drugs (e.g. serum creatinine and potassium on new ACEIs)
- Management of CVD risk with aspirin/statins (**see Cardiology 4**)
- Number of hospital admissions required?
- Compliance?
- Fluid/salt intake
- Vaccinations, e.g. influenza

Treatment options and implementation

Most patients will require loop diuretics (e.g. frusemide or bumetanide) titrated against response, to control pulmonary and peripheral oedema without dehydrating the patient's plasma compartment. Doses may be divided

ACEI (OR ARB if ACEI not tolerated due to ACEI-specific ADR)

All patients should be on an ACEI, started low and titrated upwards until maximum licensed/tolerated dose is reached. (Monitor serum creatinine, BP, and potassium as these are most common dose-limiting variables).

BETA-BLOCKERS

So long as heart failure and BP are stable, and no contraindication to beta-blocker, start carvedilol or bisoprolol in heart failure dose and titrate slowly upwards to target dose. Care to avoid hypotension or worsening the heart failure. (Patients may *temporarily* feel worse)

SPIRONOLACTONE

Introduce spironolactone in moderate or severe heart failure at a low (25 mg) dose and increase to 50 mg. Watch serum potassium, especially if taking ACEI/ARB

DIGOXIN

If still symptomatic despite above therapies add digoxin at dose appropriate for renal function. No effect on mortality but may reduce hospitalisations

OR

Start digoxin anyway if has atrial fibrillation and heart failure – high risk of stroke in this group of patients – and warfarin if appropriate

OTHER THERAPIES

Specialists may use vasodilators including nitrates and hydralazine in severe cases, or when ACEIs/ARBs not tolerated, but this is increasingly less common

Further reading: basics

- Randall MD, Neil KE. *Disease Management*. London: Pharmaceutical Press; 2003. Chapter 14: Heart failure.
- *British National Formulary*, current edn. London: Royal Pharmaceutical Society and British Medical Association. Sections 2.2: Diuretics and 2.5: ACEIs (ONLINE)

 Further reading: moving on

- Williams H, Kearney M. Heart Disease (1) Chronic heart failure. *Pharm J* 2002; 269: 325–327. (ONLINE)
- Walker R, Edwards C, eds. *Clinical Pharmacy and Therapeutics*, 3rd edn. London: Churchill-Livingstone; 2003. Chapter 19: Congestive heart failure.
- Dodds LJ, ed. *Drugs in Use*, 3rd edn. London: Pharmaceutical Press; 2003. Chapter 4: Cardiac failure.

Guidelines

- National Institute for Clinical Excellence. *Clinical Guideline 5: Management of Chronic Heart Failure in Adults in Primary and Secondary Care*. London: NICE; 2003. (ONLINE)
- Department of Health. *National Service Framework for Coronary Heart Disease*. London: Department of Health; 2000. (ONLINE)

SAQ **Self-assessment questions: Cardiology 3** (Answers on p. 39)

1. Are diuretics always the first-line treatment in congestive heart failure?
2. What monitoring is required during diuretic therapy?

3. What benefits do ACEIs offer in congestive heart failure?
4. Why do some people need to start ACEIs in hospital?
5. What monitoring is needed when initiating ACEIs?
6. What is the role of ARBs in heart failure?
7. Are beta-blockers considered safe in heart failure?
8. How do beta-blockers and spironolactone improve morbidity and mortality in heart failure?
9. Why do many patients remain undertreated?
10. How should hypertension and ischaemic heart disease be treated in congestive heart failure?

Cardiology 4 problem: the patient needs to reduce their cardiovascular risk

 Objectives of this section

The reader should be able to detail:
- the differences between primary and secondary prevention of cardiovascular disease
- the difference between the terms 'coronary heart disease' (CHD) and 'cardiovascular disease' (CVD)
- the factors that identify populations at risk of developing CVD
- the non-drug measures that can be taken to reduce CVD risk
- statins and low-dose aspirin – whom to treat and to what targets
- particular issues in heart failure, atrial fibrillation and after an MI.

Chart 2.4 Cardiology 4 problem: the patient needs to reduce their cardiovascular risk

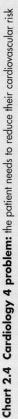

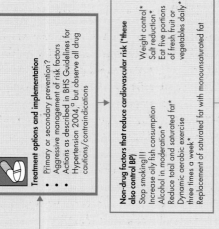

Treatment options and implementation
- Primary or secondary prevention?
- Aggressive management of risk factors
- Actions as described in BHS Guidelines for Hypertension 2004,[a] but observe all drug cautions/contraindications

Non-drug factors that reduce cardiovascular risk (*these also control BP)

Stop smoking!!!   Weight control*
Increase oily fish consumption   Salt reduction*
Alcohol in moderation*   Eat five portions
Reduce total and saturated fat*   of fresh fruit or
Dynamic aerobic exercise   vegetables daily*
three times a week*
Replacement of saturated fat with monounsaturated fat

Use of aspirin and statins
Primary prevention
Aspirin 75 mg if >50 years, BP controlled to <150/90 mmHg, and either organ damage, diabetes type 1, 10-year CVD risk of 20% or more
Statin if total cholesterol ≥3.5 mmol/L, age <80 years, and 10-year CVD risk of 20% or more, dose to targets below

Secondary prevention or in type 2 diabetes mellitus (DM)
Aspirin 75 mg in all patients unless contraindicated
Statin if total cholesterol ≥3.5 mmol/L, age <80 years, dose to targets below

Lipid targets once statins initiated
Only used if initial total cholesterol ≥3.5 mmol/L; good evidence of benefit to at least 80 years of age
Reduce total cholesterol by 25% or to <4 mmol/L, whichever gives the lower figure
or
reduce LDL cholesterol by 30% or to <2 mmol/L, whichever gives the lower figure

Special cases
Atrial fibrillation: rate control with digoxin or other therapy then warfarinise for stroke prevention
MI: need beta-blocker and ACEI as per NICE/NSF
Ischaemic stroke: may add dipyridamole SR 200 mg bd in addition to aspirin
Congestive heart failure: evidence for statin use is weaker but increasingly used
Acute coronary syndrome: aspirin + clopidogrel for 12 months, then stop clopidogrel

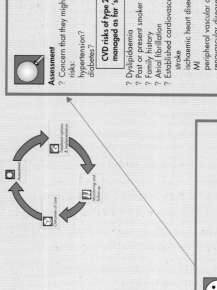

Assessment
? Concern that they might have raised cardiovascular risks:
  hypertension?
  diabetes?

CVD risks of type 2 DM are so high it should be managed as for 'secondary prevention'

? Dyslipidaemia
? Past or present smoker
? Family history
? Atrial fibrillation
? Established cardiovascular disease:
  stroke
  ischaemic heart disease
  MI
  peripheral vascular disease
  renovascular disease
? Cautions/contraindications to drug therapy: e.g. active or recent bleeding (including haemorrhagic stroke)
? Liver dysfunction or previous reaction to statins
? Excessive alcohol

Monitoring and follow-up
- Is target cholesterol being reached?
- Is BP/blood sugar tightly controlled?
- Compliance? (notoriously poor with preventive therapies)
- Have smokers stopped smoking, are supportive measures needed (nicotine replacement, support groups, etc.)?
- Non-drug measures actively repromoted?
- Adverse events (GI bleeds/muscle and liver problems?)
- Concordance in management plan: remember alternatives if one drug is not tolerated
- Date for review if not acutely unwell, new risk factors identified

Outcomes of care
The patient will:
- have a reduced risk of developing CVD or death from established CVD
- have the lowest chance possible of suffering adverse drug events from preventive therapies

[a]Williams B, Poulter NR, Brown MJ et al. British Hypertension Society guidelines for hypertension management 2004: summary. BMJ 2004; 328: 634–640.

Further reading: basics

- Williams B, Poulter NR, Brown MJ *et al.* British Hypertension Society guidelines for hypertension management 2004 (BHS-IV): summary. *BMJ* 2004: 328: 634–640. (ONLINE)
- Williams H, McRobbie D, Davies R. Primary prevention of heart disease. *Pharm J* 2003; 270: 86–88. (ONLINE)
- Stevens M, Williams H. Secondary prevention of heart disease. *Pharm J* 2002; 269: 784–786. (ONLINE)

 Further reading: moving on

- Walker R, Edwards C, eds. *Clinical Pharmacy and Therapeutics*, 3rd edn. London: Churchill-Livingstone; 2003. Chapter 22: Dyslipidaemia.

 Guidelines

- Department of Health. *National Service Framework for Coronary Heart Disease*. London: Department of Health; 2000. (ONLINE)
- National Institute for Health and Clinical Excellence. *Technology Appraisal 94. Statins for the Prevention of Cardiovascular Events*. London: NICE; 2005.
- JBS2: Joint British Societies' guidelines on prevention of cardiovascular disease in clinical practice. *Heart* 2005; 91(suppl v): V1–V52. (ONLINE)

SAQ **Self-assessment questions:
Cardiology 4** (Answers on p. 41)

1. Are the terms 'coronary heart disease' and 'cardiovascular disease' interchangeable when talking about risk prevention?
2. What is the difference between primary and secondary prevention?
3. What non-drug factors can be addressed to prevent CVD?
4. If a patient is hypertensive and has diabetes, is this relevant to CVD risk prevention?
5. Why not just give all the population over 50 years of age aspirin daily?
6. Why are there so many conflicting guidelines for statin thresholds and targets?
7. How do statins act to prevent CVD?
8. Is any particular statin preferred?
9. When a patient has had an MI, how does this affect drug treatment?
10. What action might be appropriate if a patient refuses to take their statin therapy?
11. How are post-stroke patients treated?
12. What is the role of clopidogrel in CVD prevention?
13. Should aspirin and clopidogrel ever be used together?

 **Answers to self-assessment questions:
Cardiology 1: chronic hypertension**
(p. 27)

1. What are the consequences of a prolonged elevation in blood pressure?
   In some patients, none. But raised blood pressure is associated with an increased risk of developing CVD: strokes, MI, heart failure, ischaemic heart disease and cardiac hypertrophy. In addition, other organ systems such as the eyes and kidneys can be damaged by a raised blood pressure.
2. Why is it important to maintain blood pressure within limits, even though these limits are constantly being revised?
   The published guidelines are based on evidence derived from the best available

(Continued)

morbidity and mortality data in clinical trials. Increasingly, it is known that even squeezing a few more millimetres of mercury reduction in high-risk patients such as those with diabetes will be beneficial. The variety of governmental, quasi-governmental and professional guidelines produced at different times and for different purposes may occasionally conflict in some matters.

3. **What is the difference between a target and a threshold in the management of hypertension?**

   A threshold is the point at which treatment should be initiated, and depends on the other conditions and risk factors that a patient has. A target is the level to which blood pressures should be reduced once treatment has started, and again depends on the co-morbidity and risk. Some guidelines also list an 'audit target' which, while not ideal, would satisfy audit requirements.

4. **Is there such a thing as a blood pressure that is too low?**

   Some patients in shock or dehydration have blood pressures too low to maintain cerebral and other organ perfusion, and need inotropes, fluids and other measures to increase blood pressure and so maintain circulation. In the general population, however, blood pressure should be reduced until the targets are met or until the patient complains of adverse events such as dizziness or fainting. These symptoms will usually be worse on standing ('postural hypotension') and are aggravated by ageing and drugs such as tricyclic antidepressants, diuretics and so forth. In hospitals, many nurses would temporarily omit anti-hypertensive medication either informally or in accordance with policy when systolic BP, for example, is <100 mmHg, but this should always be reported back to the medical staff.

5. **Why are people with established cardiovascular disease, diabetes or kidney damage treated at lower thresholds and to tighter targets than the rest of the population?**

   Effectively the expected benefit when compared with the cost or risks of drug therapy justifies a more aggressive approach. To treat a large number of patients with a raised blood pressure creates workload and drug costs, and exposes the patients to the inconvenience and adverse effects of drugs. In the absence of the above co-morbidity, large numbers of patients need to be treated to prevent a death – many of this group will never go on to develop CVD even if left untreated. However, diabetes mellitus (DM) carries a large risk of developing CVD, and those with established CVD are in a much higher risk group for early mortality and increased morbidity.

6. **Should non-drug measures always be tried before initiating drug therapy?**

   The non-drug measures that reduce blood pressure can be surprisingly effective. A patient may have lived with mildly elevated blood pressure for some time, and an early introduction of drug therapy may not be in their best interest. However, where blood pressure is substantially elevated, or there are risk factors for complications, a poor family history or established CVD, most doctors would wish to initiate treatment promptly. The promotion of non-drug measures is still essential as it may reduce the need for multiple-drug therapy and higher doses of antihypertensive medication.

→

7. **How should drug therapy be initiated?**

   Using algorithms such as 'ABCD' (ACEI/ARB, beta-blocker, CCB, diuretic, see Chart 2.1) (or drugs with a good evidence base and the best possible fit with co-morbidities), drug therapy should be initiated gently with careful monitoring for adverse events. Compliance should be stressed, in addition to the risks of failure to control blood pressure, and doses increased slowly. A second and third drug may be required, added in the same way. Remember, unless excessive, hypertension is not usually an immediate danger and over-rapid reduction in blood pressure may be unpleasant or dangerous for the patient.

8. **Why is the consideration of additional measures to reduce cardiovascular risk important?**

   Hypertension is only one factor contributing to the development of CVD. Lipids, smoking, hyperglycaemia, saturated and total fat intake, exercise, stress, salt and so forth all have a part to play. Reduction of blood pressure without reduction of all risk factors will not achieve the best possible outcomes and so blood pressure cannot be considered in isolation. **Cardiology 4** considers the whole issue of CVD risk.

9. **Which is the best drug with which to start treatment?**

   In the recent past beta-blockers and thiazide diuretics were still the only classes of drugs with evidence that they did not just lower BP (necessary to get a product licence) but that they also reduced CVD mortality and morbidity (demonstrated only in large and expensive multicentre clinical trials). However, most classes of drugs have now been shown to have roughly equal efficacy in this regard (alpha-blockers still lack the same evidence of benefit, and at the time of going to press were generally reserved for use where other classes were not tolerated or were insufficient). Beta-blockers and thiazide combinations seem to have a slightly higher risk of causing diabetes than newer therapies, but they are cheaper in drug-cost terms. In general, drug choice is based on co-morbidity factors and 'ABCD'-type algorithms, although the most recent NICE guidance for primary care has recommended avoiding beta-blockers as first-line choices in hypertension unless there are compelling indications – see the guidelines (ONLINE).

10. **How does co-morbidity affect drug choice by the prescriber or pharmacist?**

    This is discussed in Table 2.1, page 29, but an example of a compelling indication might be angina. Here a beta-blocker such as atenolol (or rate-limiting CCB such as diltiazem) would control both BP and the angina symptoms. In the absence of other contraindications, atenolol would be a good first choice. An example of a compelling contraindication might be asthma. Here, beta-blockers would be contraindicated because they might worsen the asthma, but any of the other classes would be acceptable.

Answers to self-assessment questions: Cardiology 2: ischaemic heart disease (p. 31)

1. **What counselling is required when supplying a patient with GTN tablets for sublingual use?**

   The tablets should be kept in a cool, dry place and used within 8 weeks of opening the bottle, to avoid using after loss of potency. If the patient has an angina attack, they should sit down and rest, one (initially) or two tablets should be placed under the tongue and allowed to dissolve. The effect will last up to 30 minutes. If the attack is not relieved, or more than three doses are needed in 15 minutes, then an ambulance should be called – it could be a more serious cardiac event. If the number of attacks for which the tablets are needed seems to be increasing, a doctor should be consulted. ADRs include flushing and headache, and can be minimised by spitting the tablet out. Tablets can be purchased at a pharmacy if supplies are needed urgently.

2. **What advantages and disadvantages does GTN spray offer over sublingual tablet formulations?**

   The shelf-life is not limited by the 8-week rule, and the formulation remains effective even if dry mouth might have prevented tablet dissolution. However, the dose cannot be 'spat out' if ADRs occur.

3. **If a patient fails to tolerate aspirin 75 mg daily, should clopidogrel be used instead?**

   Many pharmacists and doctors are surprised to learn that there is no convincing evidence that clopidogrel is better tolerated than aspirin at equivalent doses, and the evidence base for aspirin in stable angina is much better. A more rational approach in the case of dyspepsia and similar problems is to co-prescribe a proton pump inhibitor (PPI) and counsel on taking the aspirin with food.

Both drugs are equally contraindicated if the patient has an active gastrointestinal (GI) bleed.

4. **A patient is taking aspirin and atenolol 100 mg daily to control their angina, but is still getting attacks. What would the next approach be?**

   Most sources and the *BNF* suggest the addition of a dihydropyridine calcium-channel blocker (DHP-CCB) such as amlodipine or felodipine at this point. However, in the interests of monotherapy, some sources might suggest changing to a rate-limiting CCB (RLCCB) such as verapamil or diltiazem in a once-daily formulation, but most would still restrict these to patients, such as people with asthma, who cannot tolerate beta-blockers.

5. **What is the place of DHP-CCBs in therapy?**

   Most sources suggest using them mainly as add-on therapy when beta-blocker therapy is insufficient. Although most of them are licensed for monotherapy, most sources would prefer a RLCCB in these situations because there is an additional anti-anginal benefit from the rate-limiting effect, and because dihydropyridine monotherapy strangely worsens angina in a minority of patients, due to a reflex tachycardia secondary to vasodilatation. In heart failure, where neither beta-blockers nor RLCCBs may be safely used, dihydropyridines may well be the preferred therapy.

6. **Should diabetic patients, and those suffering from peripheral vascular disease, COPD or asthma avoid beta-blockers?**

   Ten years ago, all the above groups would have been unlikely to receive beta-blockers. Now patients with diabetes and less-severe peripheral vascular disease (PVD) frequently receive them where there is established CVD (as in angina) or where they have had an MI.

Careful monitoring is important to avoid worsening symptoms. However, the use of beta-blockers in airway disease carries dangers of dangerously worsening the symptoms, as does their co-prescription with RLCCBs, and therefore it is generally best left to specialists to consider for patients who continue to experience symptoms despite other therapy.

7. What is the role of nicorandil in angina therapy?

The IONA study showed symptom improvement in a large group of patients with angina on a variety of choices and combinations of therapy. However, the study did not lend itself to subgroup analysis, and therefore which anginal patients will benefit is unknown. However, the drug is well tolerated and worth considering where the usual treatment pathways have failed, usually as part of a combination therapy regime.

8. Should angina patients receive a statin therapy?

Yes, unless their cholesterol is <3.5 mmol/L. Angina is the symptom of established ischaemic heart disease and carries high risks of progression to MI and/or heart failure. A drug should be chosen that has a licence for prophylaxis of cardiac events, and the usual monitoring carried out (see **Cardiology 4**).

 Answers to self-assessment questions
Cardiology 3: heart failure (p. 33)

1. Are diuretics always the first-line treatment in congestive heart failure?

Occasionally patients' conditions will be asymptomatic except on exertion, or detectable only on echocardiography: left ventricular systolic dysfunction (LVSD). These patients will not require diuretics to clear the accumulation of fluid in the lungs and periphery. However, most patients will need loop diuretics to promote urinary excretion, and indeed the presence of loop diuretics and ACEIs on a prescription should raise the possibility of heart failure in a pharmacist's mind.

Loop diuretics can be increased to relatively high doses during acute exacerbations, or given intravenously. However, they may need to be augmented by the co-prescription of a thiazide or metolazone, a 'thiazide-like' diuretic. These act synergistically with the loop diuretic, but the strong diuresis produced needs careful monitoring to avoid dehydration and renal failure. For this reason, they are usually only added to the regime for limited periods.

2. What monitoring is required during diuretic therapy?

Patients should be weighed daily during acute periods to check how much fluid is being lost – typically a maximum loss of 500 g–1 kg (representing 0.5–1 L fluid) daily is desirable. If fluid is forced out too quickly there will be a drop in the plasma volume before the overall oedema is cleared. This hypovolaemia will lead to a drop in renal perfusion, and may even lead to renal failure, so creatinine and electrolytes should be monitored daily during initial diuretic treatment, especially if metolazone or bendroflumethiazide has been co-prescribed with the loop diuretic. Blood pressure and infusion rates of frusemide

(Continued)

should also be observed. Less frequent monitoring may be appropriate in the chronic situation.

3. **What benefits do ACEIs offer in congestive heart failure?**

   Diuretics provide symptomatic relief and prevent the patient dying from acute pulmonary oedema. But ACEIs increase survival and reduce morbidity on top of this short-term benefit. This has been well proven in many clinical trials. Add to this the substantial reduction in the development of new heart failure after an MI, and it is no surprise that all the current guidelines say that ACEIs should be started in all suitable patients, whether the heart failure is symptomatic or not.

4. **Why do some people need to start ACEIs in hospital?**

   The *BNF* lists patients who need the close supervision of a hospital ward when starting ACEIs – those over 70 years, on big doses of loop diuretics, with low sodium levels etc. This is because these patients are most likely to have mild hypovolaemia from their diuretics, and thus activation of the renin–angiotensin–aldosterone system in the kidney as a reponse. As a result, these are the patients most prone to the hypotensive effects of ACEIs when this pathway is blocked by the initiation of a drug in this class. Because of the risks of exacerbating the first-dose drop in blood pressure, the *BNF* advises that all diuretics should be stopped temporarily when initiating ACEIs, but in heart failure this is often not possible.

5. **What monitoring is needed when initiating ACEIs?**

   This is well detailed in the *BNF*. In addition to blood pressure, ACEIs can lead to hyperkalaemia, especially when the heart failure has led to a mild renal impairment. Fortunately, loop diuretics have a hypokalaemic effect, although this is a lot milder than that of thiazides. Before starting ACEIs any potassium-sparing diuretics that the patient was taking with their loop diuretic should be stopped (although very occasionally patients seem to need that combination restored). (Spironolactone is a potassium-sparing diuretic but the low doses used mean that hyperkalaemia is only rarely seen in combination with ACEIs, although monitoring is still required.) Creatinine also requires monitoring. There is a renovascular condition called bilateral renal artery stenosis (BRAS), often undiagnosed although it can be suspected if there is substantial peripheral vascular disease, especially in diabetes. In BRAS, the initiation of an ACEI or a substantial increase in dose can drop renal perfusion and lead to acute renal failure. Patients can be asked about dry cough, and any signs of haematological problems (fever, bruising, etc.) can be followed up with blood tests.

6. **What is the role of ARBs in heart failure?**

   At least one ARB is now licensed for heart failure and some trials have shown morbidity and mortality benefits from ARBs. This means that they present an alternative, possibly unlicensed, to ACEIs in heart failure. Sadly, there is a considerable overlap in adverse events and the lower risk of dry cough (often overly emphasised with ACEIs) is their major advantage at present. The greater evidence base for ACEIs, and their licensed status, means that they remain currently the first choice of therapy.

7. **Are beta-blockers considered safe in heart failure?**

   Ten years ago, beta-blockers were considered contraindicated in heart failure because of their negative inotropic effect. However, a series of trials have shown that certain beta-blockers, initiated in stable heart failure in a cautious and observed

→

manner, can add to the survival benefits of ACEIs. Careful titration upwards is needed, and dose increase must be stopped before symptoms are worsened by negative inotropy.

8. **How do beta-blockers and spironolactone improve morbidity and mortality in heart failure?**

The prevailing theory is that the reduction in cardiac output in heart failure leads to compensatory mechanisms which keep the patients asymptomatic for long periods. The sympathetic nervous system is activated to stimulate the heart and the renin–angiotensin–aldosterone system to increase blood pressure and maintain renal perfusion. Blocking these systems may reduce the work demanded of the heart and increase its overall efficiency. Beta-blockers may, however, initially worsen symptoms but patients should be encouraged to persist if possible.

9. **Why do many patients remain undertreated?**

Many patients do not have their ACEIs increased to the maximum tolerated/licensed dose, and so presumably will not demonstrate the benefits expected from clinical trials. Similarly, eligible patients are not getting started on beta-blockers and spironolactone. Many prescribers fear provoking adverse events in what is often a frail, elderly population, and the workloads involved in titrating and monitoring. In addition, established heart failure has traditionally been associated with truly shocking outcomes, and getting the message across that there are effective remedies takes time. NICE provides guidelines for heart failure stress, treating depression, encouraging exercise and healthy living, and taking a generally more positive approach to the condition.

10. **How should hypertension and ischaemic heart disease be treated in congestive heart failure?**

Hypertension is obviously best treated with ACEIs (or ARBs) at optimal doses, if they are tolerated. Thiazides are used, but if the patient is on loop diuretics they are usually not suitable for co-prescription, except for short periods. Beta-blockers and RLCCBs were traditionally not used, because of their negative inotropy (except for the specialist use of beta-blockers described above), and so there is certainly a place for DHP-CCBs, and amlodipine has been shown to be safe in heart failure in the PRAISE study. Nitrates also have an important role in treating ischaemic heart disease with concurrent heart failure.

 Answers to self-assessment questions
Cardiology 4: cardiovascular risk management (p. 35)

1. **Are the terms 'coronary heart disease' and 'cardiovascular disease' interchangeable when talking about risk prevention?**

Morbidity and mortality from CVD is essentially the sum of that from CHD and CVD (stroke/transient ischaemic attack etc.). Since the conditions have the same risk factors, CVD risk is obtained by multiplying CHD risk by 4/3. This is why the risk calculation tables at the back of the *BNF* now talk about a 20% risk of a patient developing CVD over 10 years rather than the previous 15% risk of developing CHD.

(Continued)

The patients who fall into the 'red zone' in the tables at the back of the *BNF* have this risk of 20% over 10 years. This means, in any year, that 2% (one in 50) of them will develop CVD (new angina, non-fatal stroke, non-fatal MI or death from these causes). If they already have any of these diseases, or diabetes, the tables cannot be used.

2. **What is the difference between primary and secondary prevention?**

In general, primary prevention is where risk factors exist for developing a condition and it is desired to reduce the likelihood of developing it. Secondary prevention means that the condition is already established and it is the risk of repetition, deterioration, morbidity or mortality that is being addressed. In addition to myocardial infarction, the existence of ischaemic heart disease, cerebrovascular disease (non-haemorrhagic), PVD or atherosclerotic renovascular disease justifies secondary prevention.

3. **What non-drug factors can be addressed to prevent CVD?**

These are listed in Chart 2.4 and are well described in the BHS 2004 Hypertension Guidelines. If a patient smokes, every effort should be made to persuade him or her to stop. Reduction in consumption should be praised, so long as it does not discourage further reductions to zero consumption. Details of local support services should be readily available. It may be useful to show the patient the differences between smokers and non-smokers in the colour of cardiovascular risk category in the tables at the back of the *BNF*.

4. **If a patient is hypertensive and has diabetes, is this relevant to CVD risk prevention?**

Yes, because hypertension and diabetes both raise the risk of CVD. The BHS 2004 Hypertension Guidelines suggest that seemingly healthy patients with type 2 DM have elevated cardiovascular risks to the point at which it makes sense to treat them as for secondary prevention. The tight control of both blood pressure and glycated haemoglobin is therefore essential, along with control of lipids and all other controllable risk factors.

5. **Why not just give all the population over 50 years of age aspirin daily?**

The prescribing of any drug carries risks and, for aspirin in particular, there is a risk of complications that range from dyspepsia to a major GI bleed. In the otherwise healthy population these risks will outweigh the benefits of aspirin therapy. There is some dispute over the point at which aspirin therapy should be considered more beneficial than risky, and that leads to confusion in the minds of the public. In addition blood pressure should be controlled before starting aspirin, to avoid the risk of haemorrhagic stroke.

6. **Why are there so many conflicting guidelines for statin thresholds and targets?**

The evidence base for statin use is expanding all the time, especially in subgroups of the general population. In addition, not only do statins carry risks of morbidity and mortality as aspirin does, but they are also expensive therapies. This means that, even where clinical benefit has been shown at a population level, purchasing authorities or prescribers may decide that the risks and costs are unjustified in certain patients. The expansion of statin use has been a feature of the last decade, and it seems likely that the criteria for prescription will continue to broaden. NICE guidance on statin use was published in 2005, which basically supports the BHS 2004 recommendations, although it does reflect the need to consider the patient as an individual and their needs and

→

wishes. This is relevant when consideration is given to the large numbers of patients who need to take their statins for CVD prevention to see benefits.

7. **How do statins act to prevent CVD?**
The reduction in total cholesterol and LDL-cholesterol is associated with a lower risk of atheroma. However, this is not the full story. Recent work points to a plaque stabilisation effect and even anti-arrhythmogenic properties.

8. **Is any particular statin preferred?**
Simvastatin and pravastatin were the first drugs licensed for prophylaxis of CVD (as opposed to frank hypercholesterolaemia) following large clinical trials in Scotland and Scandinavia. However, atorvastatin became popular even before the availability of outcome trial data because of a more efficient reduction in cholesterol levels, and a presumed class-protective effect. Most statins are now prescribed as prophylaxis, but not all are licensed, and it seems prudent to use licensed drugs wherever possible.

9. **When a patient has had an MI, how does this affect drug treatment?**
This is clearly secondary prophylaxis. Statin and aspirin therapy become mandatory, unless the cholesterol is low or there is a contraindication. In addition, however, NICE guidance on MI (ONLINE) advises the commencement of an ACEI and a beta-blocker, both of which have been shown to reduce mortality after MI (from progression to heart failure and prevention of further MI/arrhythmias, respectively). If a patient has established heart failure after MI, then standard beta-blocker use is

contraindicated and statins may have fewer benefits.

10. **What action might be appropriate if a patient refuses to take their statin therapy?**
This is their right. Have the benefits of statin therapy been explained to the patient, and any concerns addressed? At the end of the day, lipid reduction addresses only one risk, and aggressive control of other risks is equally important. Non-drug measures may be effective in reducing cholesterol.

11. **How are post-stroke patients treated?**
Statins and aspirin are equally indicated in ischaemic stroke for at least 12 months. In haemorrhagic stroke, the decision as to when to start/restart aspirin should be made by a specialist physician. Dipyridamole SR produces additional benefits with aspirin in non-haemorrhagic stroke. Tight BP control is important, and evidence is emerging that certain drug combinations may be preferable.

12. **What is the role of clopidogrel in CVD prevention?**
Clopidogrel is currently listed in most guidelines only as an alternative to aspirin where aspirin has not been tolerated, although the addition of a PPI is a more logical choice. It should be remembered that clopidogrel is still contraindicated if the patient is at risk of bleeding events.

13. **Should aspirin and clopidogrel ever be used together?**
At the time of writing, the only indication for this use was following acute coronary syndrome or certain invasive cardiac procedures. However, it may be that consultants may feel the combination is appropriate in certain high-risk patients.

R Respiratory medicine

The assistance of Judith Green, Principal Pharmacist–Lecturer at Wirral Hospitals NHS Trust, in the preparation of this section is gratefully acknowledged.

Introduction

In the admitting units of NHS hospitals, or in the primary care review clinic, respiratory problems will present second only to cardiology problems in incidence. Pharmacists have vital roles to play in ensuring safe and appropriate therapy in line with the most recent guidelines, to avoid premature mortality, morbidity and distress to patients.

 ## Problem 1: the patient has chronic asthma

Asthma can flare acutely in seemingly healthy young adults, reducing their respiratory function within minutes to dangerous levels. An appropriate response to the acute presentation is important, but the underlying prophylaxis in the chronic stages, based on a stepped approach to therapy, is equally important in preventing attacks.

 ## Problem 2: the patient has chronic obstructive pulmonary disease

This is most commonly due to prolonged exposure to tobacco smoke, although there are other causes. The fluctuation in the patient's airway function between acute deterioration and their normal condition is less marked than in asthma, and often disabling. Treatment aims to optimise airway function and to prevent both acute attacks and further deterioration and progression of the disease.

 ## Problem 3: the patient needs an inhaler device

In addition to making sure that the patient is receiving the right drug therapy and doses to achieve the desired outcomes, it is equally important to ensure that the local delivery of those drugs into the patient's lungs is achieved. This means that an inhaler device is supplied that not only is the most cost-effective, but also is one that the patient can and will use, whatever their age, comprehension, manual dexterity, pulmonary function or social circumstances.

The pharmacist's role

Because the management of asthma and COPD is based on clear evidence-based guidelines, there are many opportunities for pharmacists in both the hospital and community review situations to ensure that patients are appropriately managed. In addition, pharmacists are able to bring into the encounter their knowledge of the inhaler devices available, and the appropriateness of these for different patient groups. Finally, with their excellent patient communication skills they can educate the patient on inhaler technique, prevention measures and general healthcare.

Respiratory medicine 1 problem: the patient has chronic asthma

Objectives of this section

The reader should be able to detail:
- the objectives of care in asthma
- the use of evidence-based guidelines to derive thresholds and targets of treatment
- the strategy for a multidrug approach
- the importance of promotion of compliance in preventing asthma-related symptoms
- the basic treatment options available:
  — short-acting beta$_2$-agonists
  — long-acting beta$_2$-agonists
  — corticosteroids
  — methylxanthines
  — leukotriene antagonists
- monitoring required to ensure the efficacy and safety of drug therapy.

Further reading: basics

- *British National Formulary*, current edn. London: Royal Pharmaceutical Society and British Medical Association. Section 3: Respiratory system. (ONLINE)
- Randall MD, Neil KE. *Disease Management*. London: Pharmaceutical Press; 2004. Chapter 20: Respiratory diseases: asthma and chronic obstructive airways disease.

Further reading: moving on

- Walker R, Edwards C, eds. *Clinical Pharmacy and Therapeutics*, 3rd edn. London: Churchill Livingstone; 2003. Chapter 23: Asthma.

- Dodds LJ, ed. *Drugs in Use*, 3rd edn. London: Pharmaceutical Press; 2003. Chapter 11: Asthma.

Guidelines

- British Thoracic Society and Scottish Intercollegiate Guidelines Network. *British Guideline on the Management of Asthma*. London and Edinburgh: BTS and SIGN; 2004. (ONLINE)

SAQ Self-assessment questions
Respiratory medicine 1
(Answers on p. 51)

1. What causes the symptoms of asthma?
2. What are the differences between asthma and COPD?
3. What are the arguments for and against the use of combination inhaler therapy?
4. How do the BTS/Scottish Intercollegiate Guidelines Network (SIGN) guidelines (2004) for the management of asthma determine a patient's treatment?
5. A patient is taking inhaled beclometasone 200 micrograms twice daily, inhaled salmeterol 50 micrograms twice daily and inhaled salbutamol on a when-required basis. What step of the BTS/SIGN guidelines are they at, and what should be added to therapy in the case of poor control?
6. Why is counselling for patients prescribed inhaled corticosteroids important?
7. Can beta-blockers be prescribed for their usual indications if a patient also has asthma?
8. Which inhaler device should the patient have?

Chart 2.5 Respiratory 1 problem: the patient has chronic asthma

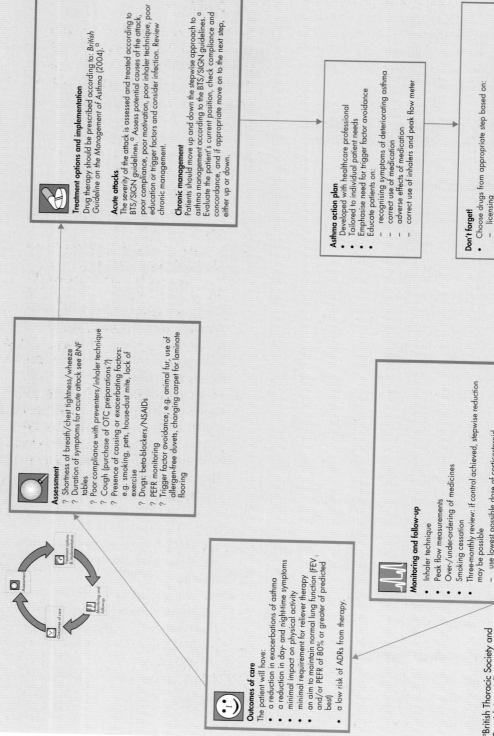

Assessment

? Shortness of breath/chest tightness/wheeze
? Duration of symptoms for acute attack see BNF tables
? Poor compliance with preventers/inhaler technique
? Cough (purchase of OTC preparations?)
? Presence of causing or exacerbating factors: e.g. smoking, pets, house-dust mite, lack of exercise
? Drugs: beta-blockers/NSAIDs
? PEFR monitoring
? Trigger factor avoidance, e.g. animal fur, use of allergen-free duvets, changing carpet for laminate flooring

Treatment options and implementation

Drug therapy should be prescribed according to: *British Guideline on the Management of Asthma* (2004).[a]

Acute attacks
The severity of the attack is assessed and treated according to BTS/SIGN guidelines. Assess potential causes of the attack, poor compliance, poor motivation, poor inhaler technique, poor education or trigger factors and consider infection. Review chronic management.

Chronic management
Patients should move up and down the stepwise approach to asthma management according to the BTS/SIGN guidelines.[a] Evaluate the patient's current position, check compliance and concordance, and if appropriate move on to the next step, either up or down.

Asthma action plan

• Developed with healthcare professional
• Tailored to individual patient needs
• Emphasise need for trigger factor avoidance
• Educate patients on:
   – recognising symptoms of deteriorating asthma
   – correct use of medication
   – adverse effects of medication
   – correct use of inhalers and peak flow meter

Don't forget!

• Choose drugs from appropriate step based on:
   – licensing
   – choice of delivery device (see **Respiratory medicine 3**)
   – evidence base.
• Emphasise the need for compliance with all preventer therapy, not just corticosteroid.
• Step up and step down therapy as appropriate – step up if poorly controlled, step down at 3-monthly intervals if well controlled

Monitoring and follow-up

• Inhaler technique
• Peak flow measurements
• Over-/under-ordering of medicines
• Smoking cessation
• Three-monthly review: if control achieved, stepwise reduction may be possible
   – use lowest possible dose of corticosteroid
   – decrease dose of inhaled steroid slowly (e.g. every 3 months) reducing dose by 20–25% each time
• For previous step, monitor chronic use of oral corticosteroids, minimise use where possible and consider osteoporosis prophylaxis

Outcomes of care

The patient will have:
• a reduction in exacerbations of asthma
• a reduction in day- and nighttime symptoms
• minimal impact on physical activity
• an aim to maintain normal lung function (FEV$_1$ and/or PEFR of 80% or greater of predicted best)
• a low risk of ADRs from therapy.

[a]British Thoracic Society and Scottish Intercollegiate Guidelines Network. *British Guideline on the Management of Asthma.* London and Edinburgh: BTS and SIGN; 2004. (ONLINE)

Respiratory medicine 2 problem: the patient has chronic obstructive pulmonary disease

Objectives of this section

The reader should be able to detail:
- the objectives of care in COPD
- the use of evidence-based guidelines to derive thresholds and targets of treatment
- the strategy for a multidrug approach
- the importance of promotion of stopping smoking
- the basic treatment options available:
  — short-acting beta$_2$-agonists
  — long-acting beta$_2$-agonists
  — antimuscarinics (anticholinergics)
  — corticosteroids
  — methylxanthines
- Monitoring required to ensure the efficacy and safety of drug therapy.

Further reading: basics

- *British National Formulary*, current edn. London: Royal Pharmaceutical Society and British Medical Association. Section 3: Respiratory system. (ONLINE)
- Randall MD, Neil KE. *Disease Management*. London: Pharmaceutical Press; 2004. Chapter 20: Respiratory diseases: asthma and chronic obstructive airways disease.

Further reading: moving on

- Walker R, Edwards C, eds. *Clinical Pharmacy and Therapeutics*, 3rd edn. London: Churchill Livingstone; 2003. Chapter 24: Chronic obstructive pulmonary disease.
- Dodds LJ, ed. *Drugs in Use*, 3rd edn. London: Pharmaceutical Press; 2003. Chapter 12: Chronic obstructive pulmonary disease.

Guidelines

- National Institute for Clinical Excellence. *Clinical Guideline 4: Management of Chronic Obstructive Pulmonary Disease in Adults in Primary and Secondary Care*. London: NICE; 2004. (ONLINE)

SAQ Self-assessment questions: Respiratory medicine 2
(Answers on p. 52)

1. What factors are responsible for the symptoms of COPD?
2. How is a patient's history of smoking calculated in pack-years?
3. What are the differences between FVC, FEV$_1$ and PEFR?
4. Is oxygen a drug?
5. Is there a difference in oxygen concentrations that should be prescribed for patients with asthma and COPD and if so, why?
6. Why are short-acting bronchodilators or 'relievers' used in COPD if they are not effective in improving lung function?
7. For each of the categories of drug listed in Table 2.2, give one or two examples and explain how lung function is improved by this therapy.

Table 2.2

Class	Example	Mode of action
Short-acting beta$_2$-agonist		
Long-acting beta$_2$-agonist		
Corticosteroid		
Methylxanthine		
Antimuscarinic		

Chart 2.6 Respiratory 2 problem: the patient has chronic obstructive pulmonary disease

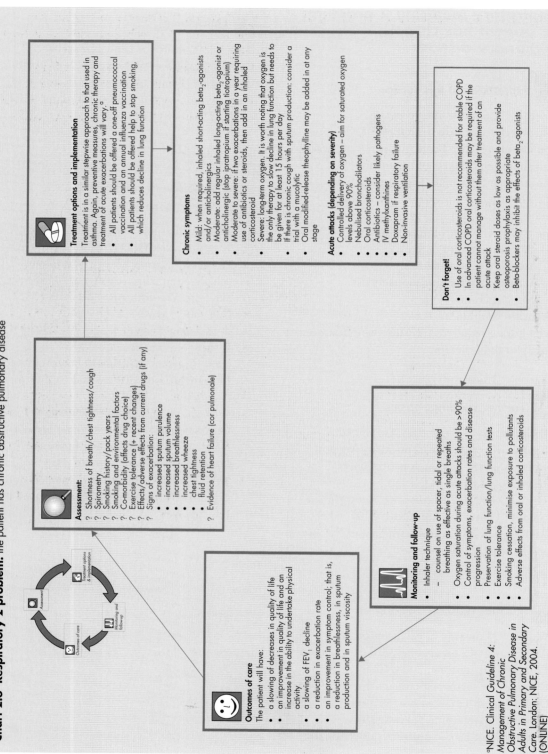

Treatment options and implementation

Treatment is in a similar stepwise approach to that used in asthma. Again, preventive measures, chronic therapy and treatment of acute exacerbations will vary.[a]

- All patients should be offered a one-off pneumococcal vaccination and an annual influenza vaccination
- All patients should be offered help to stop smoking, which reduces decline in lung function

Chronic symptoms

- Mild: when required, inhaled short-acting beta₂-agonists and/or anticholinergics
- Moderate: add regular inhaled long-acting beta₂-agonist or anticholinergic (stop ipratropium if starting tiotropium)
- Moderate to severe: if two exacerbations in a year requiring use of antibiotics or steroids, then add in an inhaled corticosteroid
- Severe: long-term oxygen. It is worth noting that oxygen is the only therapy to slow decline in lung function but needs to be given for at least 15 hours per day
- If there is chronic cough with sputum production: consider a trial with a mucolytic
- Oral modified-release theophylline may be added in at any stage

Acute attacks (depending on severity)

- Controlled delivery of oxygen – aim for saturated oxygen levels above 90%
- Nebulised bronchodilators
- Oral corticosteroids
- Antibiotics – consider likely pathogens
- IV methylxanthines
- Doxapram if respiratory failure
- Non-invasive ventilation

Don't forget!

- Use of oral corticosteroids is not recommended for stable COPD
- In advanced COPD oral corticosteroids may be required if the patient cannot manage without them after treatment of an acute attack
- Keep oral steroid doses as low as possible and provide osteoporosis prophylaxis as appropriate
- Beta-blockers may inhibit the effects of beta₂-agonists

Assessment:

? Shortness of breath/chest tightness/cough
? Spirometry
? Smoking history/pack years
? Smoking and environmental factors
? Co-morbidity (affects drug choice)
? Exercise tolerance (+ recent changes)
? Effects/adverse effects from current drugs (if any)
? Signs of exacerbation:
   • increased sputum purulence
   • increased sputum volume
   • increased breathlessness
   • increased wheeze
   • chest tightness
   • fluid retention
? Evidence of heart failure (cor pulmonale)

Monitoring and follow-up

- Inhaler technique
  – counsel on use of spacer, tidal or repeated breathing as effective as single breaths
- Oxygen saturation during acute attacks should be >90%
- Control of symptoms, exacerbation rates and disease progression
- Preservation of lung function/lung function tests
- Exercise tolerance
- Smoking cessation, minimise exposure to pollutants
- Adverse effects from oral or inhaled corticosteroids

Outcomes of care

The patient will have:

- a slowing of decreases in quality of life
- an improvement in quality of life and an increase in the ability to undertake physical activity
- a slowing of FEV_1 decline
- a reduction in exacerbation rate
- an improvement in symptom control; that is, a reduction in breathlessness, in sputum production and in sputum viscosity

[a]NICE. Clinical *Guideline 4: Management of Chronic Obstructive Pulmonary Disease in Adults in Primary and Secondary Care.* London: NICE, 2004. (ONLINE)

Respiratory medicine 3 problem: the patient needs an inhaler device

 Objectives of this section

The reader should be able to detail:

- the types of inhaler device available
- the use of evidence-derived guidelines to influence inhaler choice
- the strategy for a multidrug approach
- the choice of an inhaler device to support the basic treatment options available
- the monitoring required for efficacy and safety of drug therapy.

 Further reading: basics

- *British National Formulary*, current edn. London: Royal Pharmaceutical Society and British Medical Association. Section 3: Respiratory system. (ONLINE)

 Further reading: moving on

- Walker R, Edwards C, eds. *Clinical Pharmacy and Therapeutics*, 3rd edn. London: Churchill Livingstone; 2003. Chapter 23: Asthma.

 Guidelines

- British Thoracic Society and Scottish Intercollegiate Guidelines Network. *British Guideline on the Management of Asthma*. London and Edinburgh: BTS and SIGN; 2004. (ONLINE)
- National Institute for Clinical Excellence. *Technology Appraisal 38: Inhaler Devices for Routine Treatment of Chronic Asthma in Older Children (aged 5–15 Years)*. London: NICE; 2002.

 Self-assessment questions: Respiratory medicine 3
(Answers on p. 53)

1. When choosing an inhaler device, which should be chosen first, the device or the drug?
2. How should the appropriate device be selected for a patient?
3. Which is more important – drug or device?
4. How should a patient be counselled about the use of a spacer device?
5. What are the differences between inhaler devices available to patients?
6. In the event of an acute asthma attack, what advice could a patient be given about using a spacer device?

Chart 2.7 Respiratory 3 problem: the patient needs an inhaler device

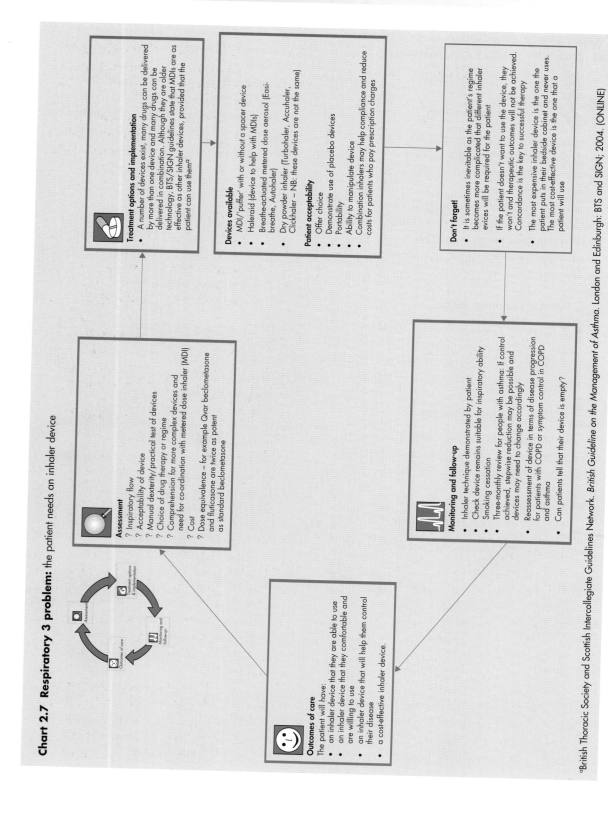

Assessment

? Inspiratory flow
? Acceptability of device
? Manual dexterity/practical test of devices
? Choice of drug therapy or regime
? Comprehension for more complex devices and need for co-ordination with metered dose inhaler (MDI)
? Cost
? Dose equivalence – for example Qvar beclometasone and fluticasone are twice as potent as standard beclometasone

Treatment options and implementation

• A number of devices exist, many drugs can be delivered by more than one device and many drugs can be delivered in combination. Although they are older technology, BTS/SIGN guidelines state that MDIs are as effective as other inhaler devices, provided that the patient can use them[a]

Devices available

• MDI/'puffer' with or without a spacer device
• Haleraid (device to help with MDIs)
• Breathe-actuated metered dose aerosol (Easi-breathe, Autohaler)
• Dry powder inhaler (Turbohaler, Accuhaler, Clickhaler – NB: these devices are not the same)

Patient acceptability

• Offer choice
• Demonstrate use of placebo devices
• Portability
• Ability to manipulate device
• Combination inhalers may help compliance and reduce costs for patients who pay prescription charges

Don't forget!

• It is sometimes inevitable as the patient's regime becomes more complicated that different inhaler devices will be required for the patient
• If the patient doesn't want to use the device, they won't and therapeutic outcomes will not be achieved. Concordance is the key to successful therapy
• The most expensive inhaler device is the one the patient puts in their bedside cabinet and never uses. The most cost-effective device is the one that a patient will use

Monitoring and follow-up

• Inhaler technique demonstrated by patient
• Check device remains suitable for inspiratory ability
• Smoking cessation
• Three-monthly review for people with asthma: if control achieved, stepwise reduction may be possible and devices may need to change accordingly
• Reassessment of device in terms of disease progression for patients with COPD or symptom control in COPD and asthma
• Can patients tell that their device is empty?

Outcomes of care

The patient will have:
• an inhaler device that they are able to use
• an inhaler device that they comfortable and are willing to use
• an inhaler device that will help them control their disease
• a cost-effective inhaler device.

[a]British Thoracic Society and Scottish Intercollegiate Guidelines Network. *British Guideline on the Management of Asthma*. London and Edinburgh: BTS and SIGN; 2004. (ONLINE)

Answers to self-assessment questions:
Respiratory medicine 1: asthma (p. 45)

1. **What causes the symptoms of asthma?**
   Asthma is caused by a mixture of bronchospasm and airway hyper-responsiveness, excessive mucus production, chronic inflammation and reversible airflow limitation. It may be triggered by allergens (dust, house-dust mite faeces, pollens etc.), pollutants, drugs and a stress response.

2. **What are the differences between asthma and COPD?**
   In asthma, airflow obstruction is variable and usually completely reversible.

   Asthma has a potentially complete response to beta$_2$-agonist use, whereas in COPD impairment of lung function is largely fixed and is only partially reversible or not reversible by bronchodilator therapy. Asthma is caused by genetic predisposition and exposure to trigger factors, whereas COPD is usually caused by smoking. Exacerbations of asthma are usually caused by environmental trigger factors rather than bacterial infection, which is the predominant cause of COPD exacerbations.

3. **What are the arguments for and against the use of combination inhaler therapy?**
   Combination therapy is more cost-effective since combination inhalers are usually cheaper than the cost of two separate inhalers. There is only one prescription charge for the patient and, since there is only one inhaler to use regularly, the patient may have improved compliance (although there is no evidence for this). There are problems with combination inhalers including a lack of flexibility in dosing, for example with Seretide in terms of salmeterol dosing. In addition, a lack of beclometasone combinations encourages the use of Seretide – one of the most potent steroids available.

4. **How do the BTS/SIGN Guidelines (2004) for the management of asthma determine a patient's treatment?**
   The BTS guidelines work on a 'step up' and 'step down' system. Where asthma is poorly controlled, a step up to a higher intensity of therapy is indicated which varies depending on which step of therapy the patient is currently on. Where asthma has been well controlled for three or more months, a step down may be indicated. The benefit of this may be to reduce the patient's exposure or need for drug therapy which can help compliance and reduce the potential for adverse effects, particularly with reference to corticosteroids, and will also reduce drug costs.

5. **A patient is taking inhaled beclometasone 200 micrograms twice daily, inhaled salmeterol 50 micrograms twice daily and inhaled salbutamol on a when-required basis. What step of the BTS/SIGN guidelines are they at, and what should be added to therapy in the case of poor control?**
   This patient is at 'step 3' of the guidelines and, in the case of poorly controlled asthma, the first response should be to increase the inhaled corticosteroid, beclometasone, from a standard dose, 200 micrograms twice a day, to a high dose, defined by the guidelines as 0.8–2 mg daily in divided doses. If this fails to control the asthma, the guidelines suggest, on a six-week sequential therapeutic trial basis, the addition of either a leukotriene antagonist, modified-release oral theophylline or modified-release oral beta$_2$-agonist.

6. **Why is counselling for patients prescribed inhaled corticosteroids important?**
   Patients need to use their inhaled corticosteroids to reduce the risk of their

(Continued)

symptoms recurring and for this reason they are termed 'preventers'. The problem with inhaled corticosteroids is that patients feel no immediate benefit, and therefore perceive them to be ineffective. Another issue is that they can cause oral thrush and sore throat which can deter patients from using their inhalers. Therefore counselling about the importance of using the device regularly, using a spacer device and rinsing of the mouth is important to prevent sore throat, hoarsness and oral candidiasis. A 'steroid card' should also be supplied for patients receiving high-dose inhaled steroids due to the risk of adrenal suppression and the need to avoid abrupt cessation of therapy.

7. **Can beta-blockers be prescribed for their indications if a patient also has asthma?**
   In short, no, unless there are compelling reasons, and under specialist supervision. See the *BNF* under contraindications for beta-blockers and the Committee on the Safety of Medicines' (CSM) warning in the *BNF* for further details.

8. **Which inhaler device should the patient have?**
   Choice of device is covered in **Respiratory medicine 3**. However, the most effective device in terms of cost and therapeutic outcomes is the one that the patient can and will use.

Answers to self-assessment questions:
Respiratory medicine 2: chronic obstructive pulmonary disease (p. 47)

1. **What factors are responsible for the symptoms of COPD?**
   Symptoms of COPD include cough, sputum production and dyspnoea on exertion. Smoking, including passive smoking, is the number one cause, but environmental causes, pollution or alpha$_1$-antitrypsin deficiency may be responsible in some cases.

2. **How is a patient's history of smoking calculated in pack-years?**
   One packet of 20 cigarettes smoked every day for one year equals one pack-year. Total pack-years equals the average number of cigarettes smoked each day, divided by 20, and multiplied by the number of years smoked for. This measurement is useful for estimating the degree of smoking history of the patient.

3. **What are the differences between FVC, FEV$_1$ and PEFR?**

FVC is the forced vital capacity, FEV$_1$ is the forced expiratory volume in 1 second while PEFR is the peak expiratory flow rate
   FEV$_1$ and the FEV$_1$/FVC ratio tend to be used for diagnosis and assessment of progression of COPD and these patients tend to have a decrease in both. PEFR tends to be used in asthma to measure severity of airway obstruction. PEFR is less useful in the assessment of COPD because it measures air flow in larger airways. Since COPD is a disease of smaller airways, PEFR is not a good indicator of disease severity, but may be used to measure a response to treatment.

4. **Is oxygen a drug?**
   Oxygen should be prescribed as a drug since it meets all the criteria for a drug, and it can kill patients if used inappropriately.

5. **Is there a difference in oxygen concentrations that should be prescribed for patients with asthma and COPD and, if so, why?**
   Oxygen should be prescribed in high concentrations for asthma, and up to 100%

 →

oxygen may be required in the acute situation. For patients with COPD, oxygen should normally be prescribed at concentrations of between 24% and 28%.

In healthy individuals, respiratory drive is due to high CO_2 blood concentrations. Some COPD patients become used to high CO_2 concentrations and respiration becomes partly driven by hypoxia. Thus, if a patient dependent on hypoxia for respiratory drive is given high-strength oxygen, this drive is reduced and the patient may become acidotic and die.

6. **Why are short-acting bronchodilators or 'relievers' used in COPD if they are not effective in improving lung function?**
Beta-agonists are not effective in improving objective measures of lung function, but are effective in relieving subjective or symptomatic aspects of breathlessness.

7. **For each of the categories of drug listed in Table 2.2, give one or two examples and explain how symptoms are improved by this therapy.**
See Table 2.3.

Table 2.3

Class	Example	Mode of action
Short-acting beta$_2$-agonist	Salbutamol, terbutaline	Relaxes airway smooth muscle
Long-acting beta$_2$-agonist	Salmeterol, formoterol	Relaxes airway smooth muscle
Corticosteroid	Beclometasone, fluticasone, budesonide	Anti-inflammatory effect
Methylxanthine	Aminophylline, theophylline	Relaxes bronchial smooth muscle by inhibition of phosphodiesterase. Increases the rate and force of cardiac contraction. Increases diaphragmatic contraction and strength of respiratory muscles
Antimuscarinic	Ipratropium, tiotropium	Inhibits the bronchoconstrictory action of acetylcholine at vagal nerve endings

 Answers to self-assessment questions: Respiratory medicine 3: inhaler device selection (p. 49)

1. **When choosing an inhaler device, which should be chosen first, the device or the drug?**
Ordinarily the drug or drug class should be chosen first since therapy should be selected based on the stepwise approaches to treating asthma and COPD. Remember there may be more than one drug and, with more than one device for each class of drug in the stepwise approach, this may widen your choice of inhaler devices. For example, a salmeterol metered dose inhaler (MDI) or a salmeterol Accuhaler may be used as an alternative to a formoterol Turbohaler. For some drugs there are no alternatives, for example, ipratropium is the only short-acting antimuscarinic drug available, and is presented only as an MDI.

2. **How should the appropriate device be selected for a patient?**
Choose a starting point, usually with cost-effectiveness in mind; MDIs offer a good starting point due to their low acquisition

(Continued)

costs. The range of devices available and the range of drugs that they cover should also be considered. Assess the patient's likely inspiratory flow; this is really important for dry powder and breath-actuated inhalers. If these flow rates are too low, breath-actuated inhalers may not be activated, or for some dry powder inhalers' flow rates may be insufficient to achieve optimal lung deposition. Make an educated guess as to what is going to be practical and what is not. Does the patient need to carry the inhaler around or will it be required only at the bedside? If the inhaler is to be used in public, is it acceptable for the patient?

3. **Which is more important – drug or device?**
Neither – they are both equally important. There is no point choosing the right drug if you can't get the drug into the patient. Similarly, there is no point choosing a device if it doesn't offer the appropriate therapeutic choices.

4. **How should a patient be counselled about the use of a spacer device?**
The spacer should be compatible with the MDI being used. The drug should be administered by repeated single actuations of the MDI into the spacer, each followed by inhalation. There should be a minimal delay between MDI actuation and inspiration. Tidal breathing, that is, breathing in and out four or five times without holding each breath, is as effective as holding single breaths. Spacers should be washed monthly in warm soapy water and allowed to drip dry. The use of tea-towels to dry large-volume spacer devices causes the adhesion of drug to the spacer device walls. Spacers should be changed every 6–12 months depending on the device.

5. **What are the differences between inhaler devices available to patients?**
Two basic categories exist: the dry powder inhaler and aerosol devices. Dry powder inhalers are all breath actuated; aerosol inhalers can be divided into MDIs or breath-actuated inhalers. Clearly MDIs require more complex co-ordination, whereas breath-actuated inhalers do not as long as the patient has the inspiratory flow required to activate the device.

6. **In the event of an acute asthma attack, what advice could a patient be given about using a spacer device?**
If the patient is acutely unwell and does not have access to a nebuliser device, the patient can use 20 puffs of salbutamol into a spacer device, using an MDI, and inhaling using a tidal breathing technique.

ER Endocrinology and rheumatology

Chapter contents

The assistance of Fiona McFarlane, Teacher–Practitioner Pharmacist at Wirral Hospitals NHS Trust, in the preparation of this section is gratefully acknowledged.

Introduction

Pharmacists working in general medicine will come across patients suffering from a wide range of disease states, but diabetes mellitus (DM) and rheumatology are among those where advances in pharmacotherapy have revolutionised care in recent years.

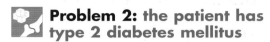 Problem 1: the patient has type 1 diabetes mellitus

Although less common than type 2 DM, the complete failure of endogenous insulin secretion, usually in childhood, was always fatal until the availability of animal insulins in the 1920s. The consequences of this condition can still be devastating, and good pharmaceutical care is necessary to avoid problems arising.

Problem 2: the patient has type 2 diabetes mellitus

The true scale and consequences of the epidemic of this condition, which is arising in the developed world, are becoming apparent. Patients should be treated to the most recent targets, if these can be tolerated. The cardiovascular risk associated with both type 1 and type 2 diabetes is considered so high that the most recent UK hypertension and lipid guidelines demand that all relevant prevention measures are adopted, even in the apparently healthy patient.

Problem 3: the patient has rheumatoid arthritis

Rheumatoid arthritis (RA) is best considered as an aggressive, systemic, auto-immune disease that involves a variety of organ systems and can devastate sufferers' lives. Treatment is intended to induce a remission in the disease process, but the drugs used may potentially have serious adverse effects and close monitoring is needed. Changes in therapy are often required over the course of many decades because of flares of the condition or a development of intolerance to a particular drug.

The pharmacist's role

In chronic, lifelong conditions such as DM and RA, pharmacists must act to ensure that the most appropriate treatments are used, targets for treatment achieved and adverse effects kept to a minimum. Concordance is important to maintain compliance and good partnerships between patients and carers.

Endocrinology and rheumatology 1 problem: the patient has type 1 diabetes mellitus

 Objectives of this section

The reader should be able to detail:

- the objectives of care in patients with type 1 DM
- the importance of promotion of healthy lifestyle choices
- the use of evidence-based guidelines to derive thresholds and targets of treatment
- the role of drug therapy in DM management
- a list of factors influencing choice of insulin and delivery system
- the complications of DM and how these can be treated
- the basic treatment options available:
  — insulin
  — ACEIs and antihypertensives
  — lipid-lowering agents/aspirin
- monitoring required to ensure the efficacy and safety of drug therapy.

 Further reading: basics

- *British National Formulary*, current edn. London: Royal Pharmaceutical Society and British Medical Association. Section 6.1: Drugs used in diabetes. (ONLINE)
- Randall MD, Neil KE. *Disease Management*. London: Pharmaceutical Press; 2004. Chapter 33: Diabetes mellitus.

 Further reading: moving on

- Walker R, Edwards C, eds. *Clinical Pharmacy and Therapeutics*, 3rd edn. London: Churchill Livingstone; 2003. Chapter 42: Diabetes mellitus.
- The Diabetes Control and Complications Trial Research Group. The effect of intensive treatment of diabetes on the development and progression of long-term complications in insulin-dependent diabetes mellitus. *N Engl J Med* 1993; 329: 977–986.

 Guidelines

- National Institute for Clinical Excellence. *Clinical Guideline 15: Type 1 Diabetes: Diagnosis and management of type 1 diabetes in adults*. London: NICE; 2004. (ONLINE)
- National Institute for Clinical Excellence. *Technology Appraisal 53: The Clinical Effectiveness and Cost Effectiveness of Long Acting Insulin Analogues for Diabetes*. London: NICE; 2002. (ONLINE)
- JBS 2. Joint British Societies' guidelines on prevention of cardiovascular disease in clinical practice. Heart 2005: 91 (supplement v), v1–v51. (ONLINE)

 Self-assessment questions: Endocrinology and rheumatology 1
(Answers on p. 63)

1. What are the World Health Organization (WHO) diagnostic criteria for DM?
2. What types of insulin are available?
3. What are insulin analogues?
4. What factors affect insulin requirements?
5. What are the major complications of poorly controlled DM in the long term? What is the cause of these complications?
6. What are the targets for the management of blood pressure in patients with type 1 DM?
7. What are the recommendations for the management of blood lipids in patients with type 1 DM?
8. When should antiplatelet therapy be initiated in patients with type 1 DM?
9. Describe the approaches to managing CVD in diabetes.
10. What are the targets for haemoglobin A_{1c} (HbA$_{1c}$) in type 1 DM?
11. When is it appropriate to use insulin glargine?

Chart 2.8 Endocrinology and rheumatology 1 problem: the patient has type 1 diabetes mellitus

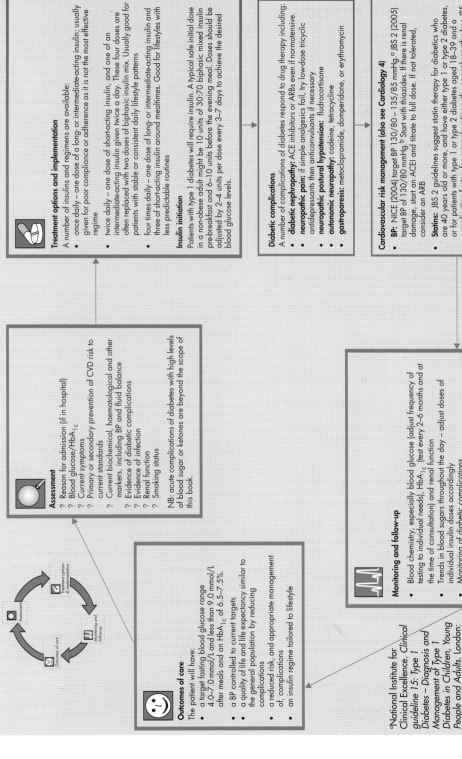

Assessment

? Reason for admission (if in hospital)
? Blood glucose/HbA₁c
? Current symptoms
? Primary or secondary prevention of CVD risk to current standards
? Current biochemical, haematological and other markers, including BP and fluid balance
? Evidence of diabetic complications
? Evidence of infection
? Renal function
? Smoking status

NB: acute complications of diabetes with high levels of blood sugar or ketones are beyond the scope of this book.

Treatment options and implementation

A number of insulins and regimens are available:

- once daily – one dose of a long- or intermediate-acting insulin; usually given for poor compliance or adherence as it is not the most effective regime
- twice daily – one dose of short-acting insulin, and one of an intermediate-acting insulin given twice a day. These four doses are often replaced with two doses of biphasic insulin mix. Usually good for patients with stable or consistent daily lifestyle patterns
- four times daily – one dose of long- or intermediate-acting insulin and three of short-acting insulin around mealtimes. Good for lifestyles with less predictable routines

Insulin initiation

Patients with type 1 diabetes will require insulin. A typical safe initial dose in a non-obese adult might be 10 units of 30:70 biphasic mixed insulin pre-breakfast and 6–10 units before the evening meal. Doses should be adjusted by 2–4 units per dose every 3–7 days to achieve the desired blood glucose levels.

Diabetic complications

A number of complications of diabetes respond to drug therapy including:

- **diabetic nephropathy:** ACE inhibitors or ARBs even if normotensive.
- **neuropathic pain:** if simple analgesics fail, try low-dose tricyclic antidepressants then anticonvulsants if necessary
- **neuropathic postural hypotension:** fludrocortisone
- **autonomic neuropathy:** codeine, tetracycline
- **gastroparesis:** metoclopramide, domperidone, or erythromycin

Cardiovascular risk management (also see Cardiology 4)

- **BP:** NICE (2004) target BP 130/80 – 135/85 mmHg,ᵃ JBS 2 (2005) target BP of 130/80 mmHg.ᵇ Start with thiazides. If there is renal damage, start an ACEI and titrate to full dose. If not tolerated, consider an ARB
- **Statins:** JBS 2 guidelines suggest statin therapy for diabetics who are 40 years old or more, and have either type 1 or type 2 diabetes, or for patients with type 1 or type 2 diabetes aged 18–39 and a complicating factor, for example retinopathy or nephropathy (see JBS 2 for further details)ᵇ
- **Aspirin:** JBS 2 guidelines suggest aspirin for patients with established cardiovascular disease and selected patients with diabetes that are 50 years of age or older, or who are younger but have had the disease for 10 years or more, or who are already receiving treatment for hypertension, once blood pressure has been controlled to <150 mmHg systolic and <90 mmHg diastolicᵇ

Outcomes of care

The patient will have:

- a target fasting blood glucose range 4.0–7.0 mmol/L and less than 9.0 mmol/L after meals and an HbA₁c of 6.5–7.5%.
- a BP controlled to current targets
- a quality of life and life expectancy similar to the general population by reducing complications
- a reduced risk, and appropriate management of, complications
- an insulin regime tailored to lifestyle

Monitoring and follow-up

- Blood chemistry, especially blood glucose (adjust frequency of testing to individual needs), HbA₁c (test every 2–6 months and at the time of consultation) and renal function
- Trends in blood sugars throughout the day – adjust doses of individual insulin doses accordingly
- Monitoring of diabetic complications
- Patient-reported ADRs
- Counsel on:
  – action on hypoglycaemic episodes
  – importance of compliance
  – need for lifestyle changes
  – smoking cessation and other cardiovascular risk measures
  – storage of insulin and disposal of injection paraphernalia

ᵃNational Institute for Clinical Excellence. *Clinical guideline 15: Type 1 Diabetes – Diagnosis and Management of Type 1 Diabetes in Children, Young People and Adults.* London: NICE, 2004. (ONLINE)
ᵇJBS 2. Joint British Societies' Guidelines on Prevention of Cardiovascular Disease in Clinical Practice. *Heart* 2005; 91 (suppl V), v1–v51. (ONLINE)

Endocrinology and rheumatology 2 problem: the patient has type 2 diabetes mellitus

 Objectives of this section

The reader should be able to detail:
- the differences between type 1 and type 2 DM
- the objectives of care in patients with type 2 DM
- the importance of promotion of healthy lifestyle choices
- the use of evidence-based guidelines to derive thresholds and targets of treatment
- the role of drug therapy in DM management
- the factors influencing choice of insulin and oral hypoglycaemics
- complications of DM and how these can be treated
- the basic treatment options available:
  — oral hypoglycaemics
  — insulin
  — lipid-lowering agents/aspirin
- ACEIs and other antihypertensives
- monitoring required for efficacy and safety of drug therapy.

 Further reading: basics

- *British National Formulary*, current edn. London: Royal Pharmaceutical Society and British Medical Association. Section 6.1: Drugs used in diabetes. (ONLINE)
- Randall MD, Neil KE. *Disease Management*. London: Pharmaceutical Press; 2004. Chapter 33: Diabetes mellitus.
- National Prescribing Centre. Drug management of type 2 diabetes: summary. *MeReC Bulletin* 2004; 15: 1–4. (ONLINE)

 Further reading: moving on

- Walker R, Edwards C, eds. *Clinical Pharmacy and Therapeutics*, 3rd edn. London: Churchill Livingstone; 2003. Chapter 42: Diabetes mellitus.
- Dodds LJ, ed. *Drugs in Use*, 3rd edn. London: Pharmaceutical Press; 2003. Chapter 25: Type 2 diabetes mellitus.

 Guidelines

- National Institute for Clinical Excellence. *Clinical Guideline H: Type 2 Diabetes – Management of Blood Pressure and Blood Lipids*. London: NICE; 2002. (ONLINE)
- National Institute for Clinical Excellence. *Clinical Guideline F: Management of Type 2 Diabetes – Renal Disease Prevention and Early Management*. London: NICE; 2002. (ONLINE)
- National Institute for Clinical Excellence. *Clinical Guideline G: Management of Type 2 Diabetes – Managing Blood Glucose Levels*. London: NICE; 2002. (ONLINE)
- National Institute for Clinical Excellence. *Technology Appraisal 63: Full Guidance on the use of Glitazones for the Treatment of Type 2 Diabetes*. London: NICE; 2003. (ONLINE)

 Self-assessment questions: Endocrinology and rheumatology 2
(Answers on p. 64)

1. What is the difference between type 1 and type 2 DM?
2. What were the key findings of the UK Prospective Diabetes Study (UKPDS)?
3. What are the targets for the management of blood pressure in patients with type 2 DM, and which drugs should be used?
4. What are the recommendations for the management of blood lipids in patients with type 2 DM?
5. When should antiplatelet therapy be initiated in patients with type 2 DM?

(Questions continued on page 60)

Chart 2.9   Endocrinology and rheumatology 2 problem: the patient has type 2 diabetes mellitus

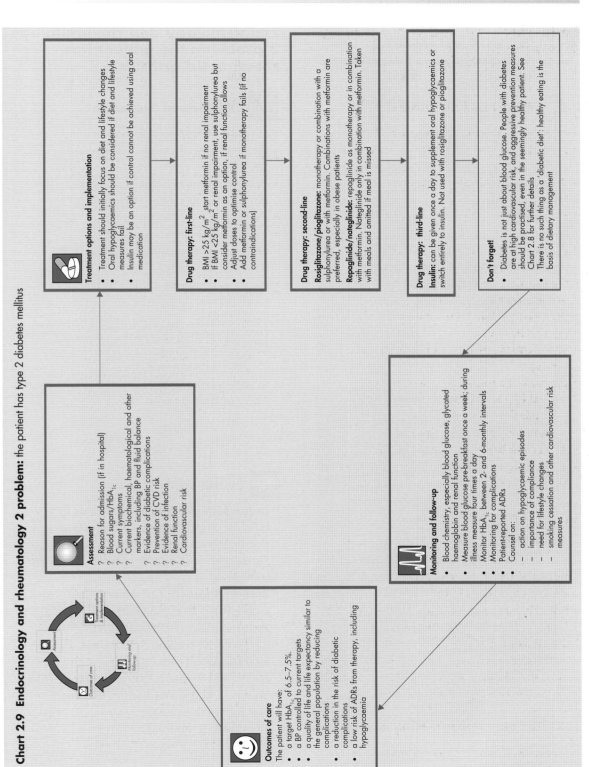

Assessment

? Reason for admission (if in hospital)
? Blood sugars/HbA₁c
? Current symptoms
? Current biochemical, haematological and other markers, including BP and fluid balance
? Evidence of diabetic complications
? Prevention of CVD risk
? Evidence of infection
? Renal function
? Cardiovascular risk

Treatment options and implementation

- Treatment should initially focus on diet and lifestyle changes
- Oral hypoglycaemics should be considered if diet and lifestyle measures fail
- Insulin may be an option if control cannot be achieved using oral medication

Drug therapy: first-line

- BMI >25 kg/m² start metformin if no renal impairment
- If BMI <25 kg/m² or renal impairment, use sulphonylurea but consider metformin as an option, if renal function allows
- Adjust doses to optimise control
- Add metformin or sulphonylurea if monotherapy fails (if no contraindications)

Drug therapy: second-line

Rosiglitazone/pioglitazone: monotherapy or combination with a sulphonylurea or with metformin. Combinations with metformin are preferred, especially in obese patients
Repaglinide/nateglinide: repaglinide as monotherapy or in combination with metformin. Nateglinide only in combination with metformin. Taken with meals and omitted if meal is missed

Drug therapy: third-line

Insulin: can be given once a day to supplement oral hypoglycaemics or switch entirely to insulin. Not used with rosiglitazone or pioglitazone

Don't forget!

- Diabetes is not just about blood glucose. People with diabetes are at high cardiovascular risk, and aggressive prevention measures should be practised, even in the seemingly healthy patient. See Chart 2.8 for further details
- There is no such thing as a 'diabetic diet': healthy eating is the basis of dietary management

Monitoring and follow-up

- Blood chemistry, especially blood glucose, glycated haemoglobin and renal function
- Measure blood glucose pre-breakfast once a week; during illness measure four times a day
- Monitor HbA₁c between 2- and 6-monthly intervals
- Monitoring for complications
- Patient-reported ADRs
- Counsel on:
  - action on hypoglycaemic episodes
  - importance of compliance
  - need for lifestyle changes
  - smoking cessation and other cardiovascular risk measures

Outcomes of care

The patient will have:
- a target HbA₁c of 6.5–7.5%.
- a BP controlled to current targets
- a quality of life and life expectancy similar to the general population by reducing complications
- a reduction in the risk of diabetic complications
- a low risk of ADRs from therapy, including hypoglycaemia

Self-assessment questions:
Endocrinology and rheumatology 2
(Continued)

6. Describe the approaches to managing CVD in DM.
7. What are the indications for insulin in type 2 DM?
8. When is it appropriate to use insulin glargine in type 2 DM?
9. Why is metformin a good choice in type 2 DM?
10. When should glitazones be used in type 2 DM?
11. How does each class of oral hypoglycaemic agent act to control blood glucose levels (use Table 2.4)?

Table 2.4

Drug	Mode of action
Biguanides: metformin	

Sulphonylureas:
  gliclazide
  glipizide
  tolbutamide
  NB:
  glibenclamide long
  acting and rarely
  used now	

Glitazones:
  rosiglitazone
  pioglitazone	

Prandial glucose
regulators:
  repaglinide
  nateglinide	

Alpha-glucosidase inhibitors: acarbose	

Endocrinology and rheumatology 3 problem: the patient has rheumatoid arthritis

 Objectives of this section

The reader should be able to detail:
- the objectives of care in patients with RA
- the use of evidence-based guidelines to derive thresholds and targets of treatment
- the role of drug therapy in RA
- The factors influencing choice of disease-modifying antirheumatic drug (DMARD) therapy
- the basic treatment options available:
  — analgesia
  — DMARDs
  — corticosteroids
  — anti-TNF α agents
  — osteoporosis prophylaxis
- monitoring required to ensure the efficacy and safety of drug therapy.

 Further reading: basics

- *British National Formulary*, current edn. London: Royal Pharmaceutical Society and British Medical Association. Section 10.1: Drugs used in rheumatic diseases and gout. (ONLINE)
- Buch M, Emery P. The aetiology and pathogenesis of rheumatoid arthritis. *Hosp Pharm* 2002; 9: 5–10. (ONLINE)
- Bayraktar A, Hudson S, Watson A, Fraser S. Pharmaceutical care (7): arthritis. *Pharm J* 2000; 264: 57–68. (ONLINE)
- Young A. Rheumatoid arthritis: current approaches to management. *Prescriber* 2004; 15: 48–55. (ONLINE)

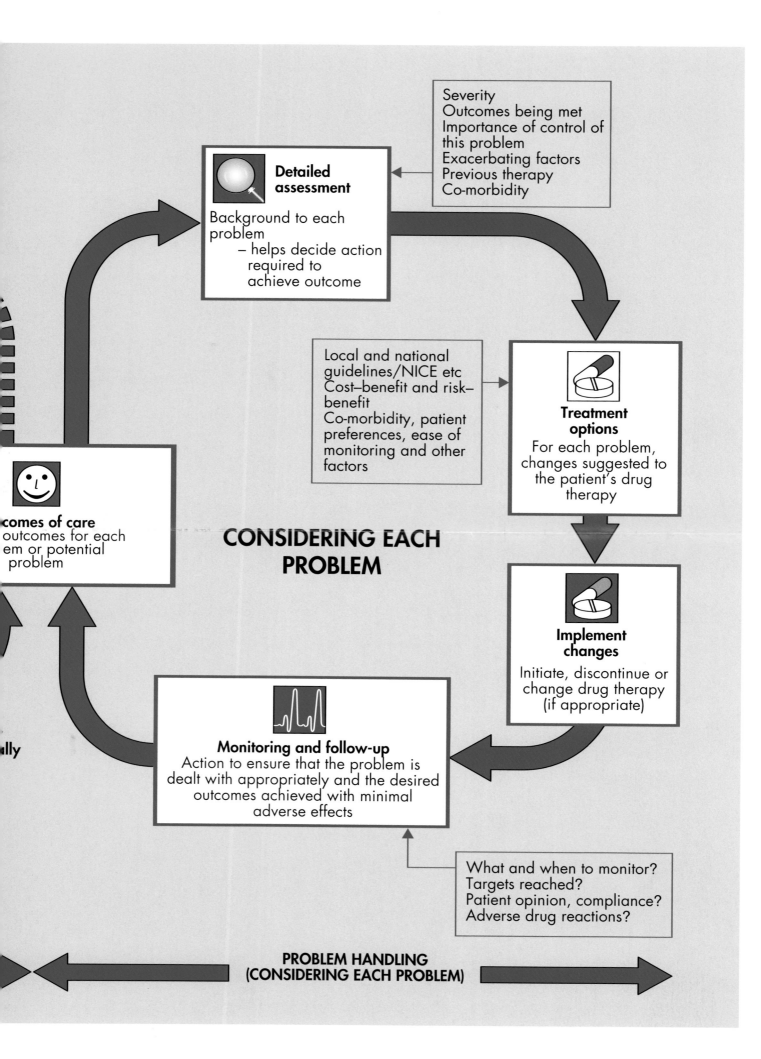

Detailed assessment

Background to each problem
– helps decide action required to achieve outcome

Severity
Outcomes being met
Importance of control of this problem
Exacerbating factors
Previous therapy
Co-morbidity

Local and national guidelines/NICE etc
Cost–benefit and risk–benefit
Co-morbidity, patient preferences, ease of monitoring and other factors

Treatment options
For each problem, changes suggested to the patient's drug therapy

comes of care
outcomes for each
em or potential
problem

CONSIDERING EACH PROBLEM

Implement changes
Initiate, discontinue or change drug therapy (if appropriate)

Monitoring and follow-up
Action to ensure that the problem is dealt with appropriately and the desired outcomes achieved with minimal adverse effects

What and when to monitor?
Targets reached?
Patient opinion, compliance?
Adverse drug reactions?

lly

**PROBLEM HANDLING
(CONSIDERING EACH PROBLEM)**

Chart 1.1 The pharmaceutical care cycle

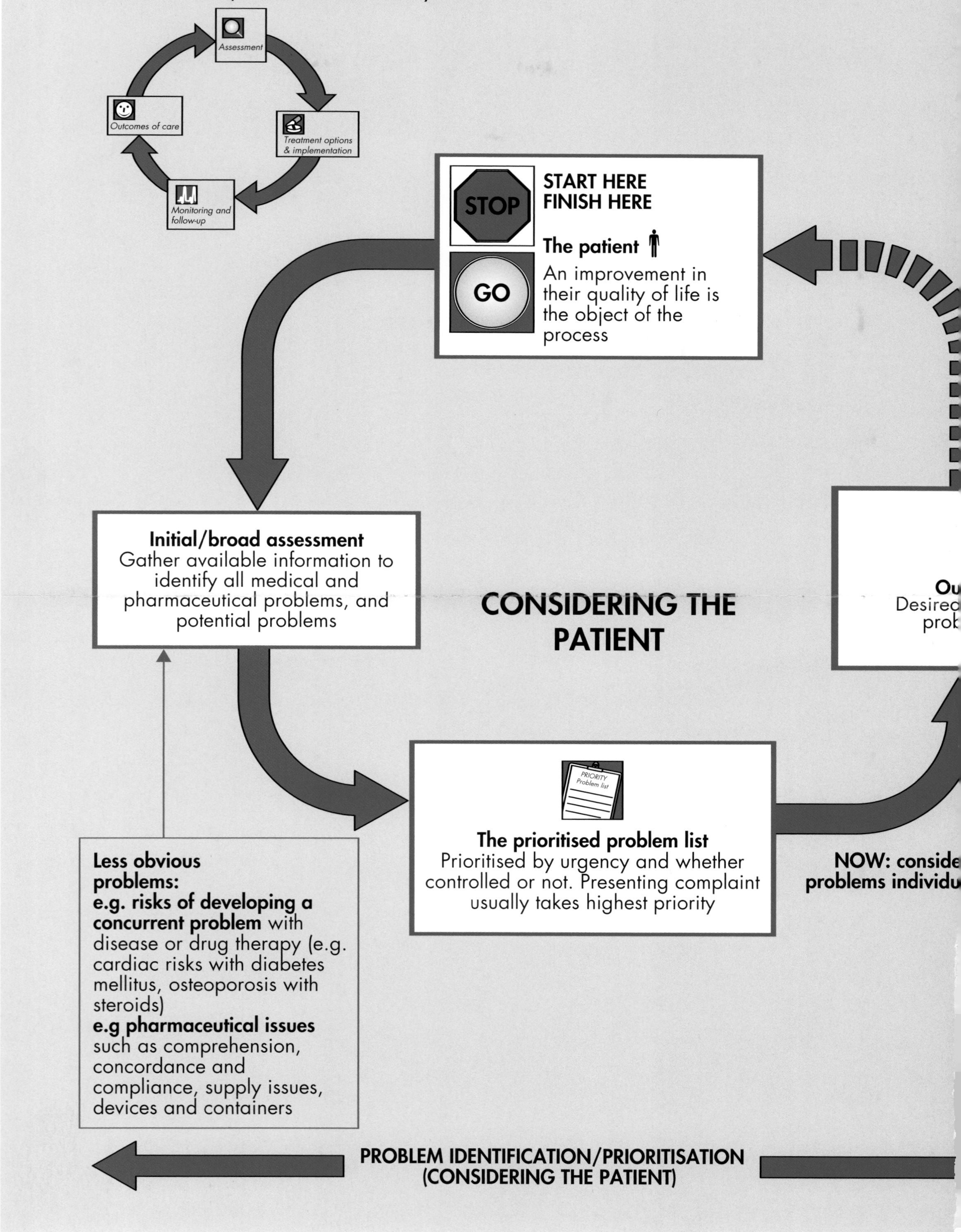

Assessment

Outcomes of care

Treatment options
& implementation

Monitoring and
follow-up

**START HERE
FINISH HERE**

STOP

The patient 🚹
An improvement in
their quality of life is
the object of the
process

GO

**CONSIDERING THE
PATIENT**

Initial/broad assessment
Gather available information to
identify all medical and
pharmaceutical problems, and
potential problems

Ou
Desire
prob

**Less obvious
problems:
e.g. risks of developing a
concurrent problem** with
disease or drug therapy (e.g.
cardiac risks with diabetes
mellitus, osteoporosis with
steroids)
e.g pharmaceutical issues
such as comprehension,
concordance and
compliance, supply issues,
devices and containers

PRIORITY
Problem list

The prioritised problem list
Prioritised by urgency and whether
controlled or not. Presenting complaint
usually takes highest priority

NOW: conside
problems individu

**PROBLEM IDENTIFICATION/PRIORITISATION
(CONSIDERING THE PATIENT)**

Further reading: moving on

- Walker R, Edwards C, eds. *Clinical Pharmacy and Therapeutics*, 3rd edn. London: Churchill Livingstone; 2003. Chapter 51: Rheumatoid arthritis and osteoarthritis.
- Dodds LJ, ed. *Drugs in Use*, 3rd edn. London: Pharmaceutical Press; 2003. Chapter 26: Rheumatoid arthritis.
- Green CF. Using anti-TNF α technology to treat rheumatoid arthritis. *Hosp Pharm* 2004; 11: 286–291. (ONLINE)
- Parkinson S, Alldred A. Drug regimens for rheumatoid arthritis. *Hosp Pharm* 2002; 9: 11–15. (ONLINE)
- NPSA: Patient safety alert no. 13: Improving compliance with oral methotrexate guidelines. At: www.npsa.nhs.uk/site/media/documents/1808_Alert.pdf (ONLINE)

 Guidelines

- National Institute for Clinical Excellence. *Technology Appraisal 36: The Clinical Effectiveness and Cost Effectiveness of Etanercept and Infliximab for Rheumatoid Arthritis and Juvenile Poly-articular Idiopathic Arthritis*. London: NICE; 2002. (ONLINE)
- National Institute for Clinical Excellence. *Technology Appraisal 72: The Clinical Effectiveness and Cost Effectiveness of Anakinra for Rheumatoid Arthritis*. London: NICE; 2003. (ONLINE)

SAQ Self-assessment questions:
Endocrinology and rheumatology 3
(Answers on p. 67)

1. What are the causes of RA?
2. What should be taken into consideration when prescribing NSAIDs?
3. What is the role of cyclo-oxygenase 2 (COX-2) inhibitors in the management of RA?
4. At what stage should DMARDs be initiated in RA patients?
5. Why is patient counselling important with DMARDs?
6. What counselling points should be covered in patients receiving DMARDs?
7. What advantages does parenteral methotrexate have over oral therapy?
8. Which biological drugs are available, and what are the differences between them?
9. What are the differences between the biological therapies in terms of dosing (Table 2.5)?
10. How can pharmacists help RA patients with compliance?
11. What options exist for the treatment of neuropathic pain in RA?

Table 2.5

Drug	Nature of drug	Presentation/administration	Dosing schedule
Infliximab (Remicaide)			
Etancercept (Enbrel)			
Adalimumab (Humira)			
Anakinra (Kineret)			

Chart 2.10 Endocrinology and rheumatology 3 problem: the patient has rheumatoid arthritis

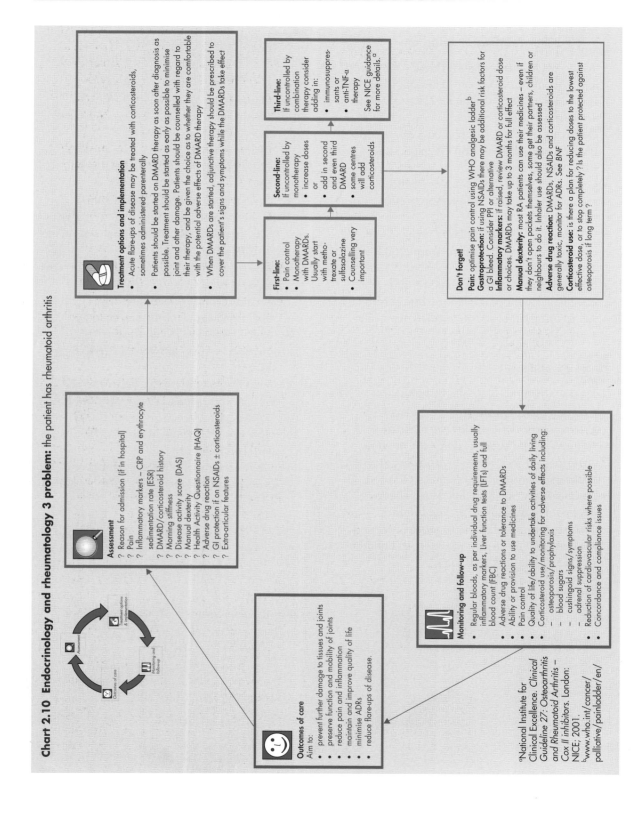

Assessment

? Reason for admission (if in hospital)
? Pain
? Inflammatory markers – CRP and erythrocyte sedimentation rate (ESR)
? DMARD/corticosteroid history
? Morning stiffness
? Disease activity score (DAS)
? Manual dexterity
? Health Activity Questionnaire (HAQ)
? Adverse drug reaction
? GI protection if on NSAIDs ± corticosteroids
? Extra-articular features

Treatment options and implementation

- Acute flare-ups of disease may be treated with corticosteroids, sometimes administered parenterally
- Patients should be started on DMARD therapy as soon after diagnosis as possible. Treatment should be started as early as possible to minimise joint and other damage. Patients should be counselled with regard to their therapy, and be given the choice as to whether they are comfortable with the potential adverse effects of DMARD therapy
- When DMARDs are started, adjunctive therapy should be prescribed to cover the patient's signs and symptoms while the DMARDs take effect

First-line:
- Pain control
- Monotherapy with DMARDs. Usually start with methotrexate or sulfasalazine
- Counselling very important

Second-line:
If uncontrolled by monotherapy
- increase doses or
- add in second and even third DMARD
- some centres will add corticosteroids

Third-line:
If uncontrolled by combination therapy consider adding in:
- immunosuppressants or anti-TNF-α therapy

See NICE guidance for more details. [a]

Monitoring and follow-up

- Regular bloods, as per individual drug requirements, usually inflammatory markers, liver function tests (LFTs) and full blood count (FBC)
- Adverse drug reactions or tolerance to DMARDs
- Ability or provision to use medicines
- Pain control
- Quality of life/ability to undertake activities of daily living
- Corticosteroid use/monitoring for adverse effects including:
  – osteoporosis/prophylaxis
  – blood sugars
  – cushingoid signs/symptoms
  – adrenal suppression
- Reduction of cardiovascular risks where possible
- Concordance and compliance issues

Outcomes of care

Aim to:
- prevent further damage to tissues and joints
- preserve function and mobility of joints
- reduce pain and inflammation
- maintain and improve quality of life
- minimise ADRs
- reduce flare-ups of disease.

Don't forget!

Pain: optimise pain control using WHO analgesic ladder [b]
Gastroprotection: if using NSAIDs there may be additional risk factors for a GI bleed. Consider PPI or alternative
Inflammatory markers: if raised, review DMARD or corticosteroid dose or choices. DMARDs may take up to 3 months for full effect
Manual dexterity: most RA patients can use their medicines – even if they don't open packets themselves, some get their partners, children or neighbours to do it. Inhaler use should also be assessed
Adverse drug reaction: DMARDs, NSAIDs and corticosteroids are generally toxic, monitor for ADRs. See BNF
Corticosteroid use: is there a plan for reducing doses to the lowest effective dose, or to stop completely? Is the patient protected against osteoporosis if long term?

[a]National Institute for Clinical Excellence. *Clinical Guideline 27: Osteoarthritis and Rheumatoid Arthritis – Cox II inhibitors.* London: NICE; 2001.
[b]www.who.int/cancer/ palliative/painladder/en/

Answers to self-assessment questions:
Endocrinology and rheumatology 1: type 1 diabetes mellitus (p. 56)

1. **What are the WHO diagnostic criteria for DM?**
   A diagnosis of DM can be made if patients have symptoms (e.g. polyuria, polydipsia or unexplained weight loss). In addition to this, patients must have a fasting glucose greater than 7.0 mmol/L, or a random venous plasma glucose concentration greater than 11.1 mmol/L. An alternative to this is the oral glucose tolerance test (OGTT) where patients with a glucose greater than 11.1 mmol/L, 2 hours after taking 75 g anhydrous glucose, are confirmed as having DM.

2. **What types of insulin are available?**
   Insulins can be classified by both source and duration of action. Human insulins are genetically engineered using either yeast or bacteria. Beef and pork insulins are purified from animal sources. Human insulin is preferred as it is less antigenic than beef or pork and is less likely to result in allergic reactions. Insulins are also categorised as short-acting or soluble insulins, intermediate-acting or isophane insulins, and long-acting or zinc suspension insulin. More recently, insulin analogues have been introduced.

3. **What are insulin analogues?**
   Modification of the amino acid sequence of the insulin peptide has led to two types of 'analogues'. Insulin lispro and insulin aspart act much faster than traditional soluble insulin and avoid the need to administer doses 30 minutes before a meal that might not arrive, which might result in hypoglycaemia. Insulin glargine and insulin detemir are long-acting insulins with a smooth activity profile that can be given once a day in both type 1 and type 2 DM.

4. **What factors affect insulin requirements?**
   Increased insulin requirements arise as a result of infection, stress, accidental or surgical trauma, puberty or pregnancy. Decreased requirements arise as a result of hepatic impairment, renal impairment or some endocrine disorders.

5. **What are the major complications of poorly controlled DM in the long term? What is the cause of these complications?**
   Microvascular complications include retinopathy, nephropathy, and autonomic, motor and sensory neuropathy. Macrovascular complications include CVD, stroke and peripheral vascular disease. Very simply, it is thought that these complications arise as a result of hyperglycaemia, which damages blood vessels, as well as a complex mixture of hormonal changes and possibly accelerated atherosclerosis.

6. **What are the targets for the management of blood pressure in patients with type 1 DM?**
   Joint British Societies' guidelines 2005 suggest a target BP of less than 130/80 mmHg in diabetic patients. NICE guidance in 2004 suggests a target of 135/85 mmHg for all patients and suggests starting therapy with a thiazide diuretic. However, for patients with confirmed kidney damage, NICE guidance suggests that all patients, including those with microalbuminuria alone, should start an ACEI and be titrated to full dose to the target of 130/80 mmHg as in the JBS 2 Guidelines. Where ACEIs are not tolerated, ARBs should be considered. Tight blood pressure control is important to reduce cardiovascular risk.

7. **What are the recommendations for the management of blood lipids in patients with type 1 DM?**
   JBS 2 guidelines suggest that statin therapy is recommended for diabetics who are 40 years

(Continued)

old or more, and have either type 1 or type 2 diabetes, or for patients with type 1 or type 2 diabetes aged 18–39 and one of the following: retinopathy, nephropathy or poor glycaemic control ($HbA_{1c} > 9\%$), elevated BP requiring antihypertensives, raised cholesterol, features of metabolic syndrome or a family history of premature cardiovascular disease. Targets of treatment are to reach a reduction of total cholesterol by 25% and LDL by 30% or to reach targets of 4 mmol/L and 2 mmol/L respectively, whichever is the greater.

8. **When should antiplatelet therapy be initiated in patients with type 1 DM?**
   JBS 2 guidelines suggest aspirin for patients with established cardiovascular disease and selected patients with diabetes who are 50 years of age or older, or who are younger but have had the disease for 10 years or more, or who are already receiving treatment for hypertension, once blood pressure has been controlled to <150 mmHg systolic and <90 mmHg diastolic.[b]

9. **Describe the approaches to managing CVD in diabetes.**
   The management of cardiovascular disease is multifactorial and includes smoking cessation, management of dyslipidaemia and hypertension, tight glycaemic control, tackling obesity, and avoiding or reducing any other risk factors.

10. **What are the targets for HbA_{1c} in type 1 DM?**
    NICE guidance suggests that the HbA_{1c} levels should be those derived from the Diabetes Control and Complications trial (DCCT) (see Endocrinology and rheumatology 1). Targets are less than 7.5% for prevention of microvascular disease and 6.5% for those at increased risk of CVD. To avoid hypoglycaemia, the individuals' preferences and experience should be considered, and advice about insulin use and available products should be arranged. With lower HbA_{1c} levels, beware of the risk of undetected or disabling hypoglycaemia and beware of compromising quality of life in pursuit of unrealistically low targets.

11. **When is it appropriate to use insulin glargine?**
    According to NICE guidance (2002), insulin glargine is an option for treating type 1 DM. In practice, it tends to be used when nocturnal hypoglycaemia is a problem on isophane insulin, morning hyperglycaemia on isophane makes day-time glucose control difficult to manage and rapid-acting insulin analogues are used for meal-time glucose control.

 Answers to self-assessment questions:
Endocrinology and rheumatology 2: type 2 diabetes mellitus (p. 58)

1. **What is the difference between type 1 and type 2 DM?**
   In type 1 DM, the patient suffers auto-immune destruction of islet cells of the pancreas. In type 2 DM, patients develop resistance to insulin and beta-cell dysfunction. It is estimated that 1.8 million of the UK population have been diagnosed with DM, of which 80% have type 2 DM. There are a further estimated 1 million cases of undiagnosed type 2 DM in the UK. Type 1 DM usually occurs at a young age, typically in lean patients. Type 1

$\longrightarrow$

DM presents in an acute manner and is subsequently static in nature. Patients are ketosis prone, and there is often a family history in about 10% of cases. Insulin treatment is mandatory. Type 2 DM usually occurs during older age, usually in obese patients and is chronic and progressive. Patients are ketosis resistant and in 30% of cases there is a positive family history. Insulin treatment is sometimes needed in type 2 DM, but is essential in type 1 DM.

2. **What were the key findings of the UK Prospective Diabetes Study (UKPDS)?**
The UKPDS showed that tight glucose control reduces both microvascular and macrovascular complications. Comparison of HbA_{1c} 7.0% versus 7.9% resulted in a 25% reduction overall in the microvascular complication rate. Comparisons between the 144/82 mmHg group and the 154/87 mmHg group showed that in the tight BP control group there was a 32% reduction in death related to DM, 44% reduction in strokes, 56% reduction in heart failure and 37% reduction in microvascular disease. However, it also showed that tight glucose control increased the incidence of attacks of hypoglycaemia.

3. **What are the targets for the management of blood pressure in patients with type 2 DM, and which drugs should be used?**
NICE guidelines in October 2002 suggest a target BP of less than 140/80 mmHg, although in the presence of microalbuminuria or proteinuria, this target BP drops to below 135/75 mmHg. More recent guidance from the JBS 2 guidelines (2005) suggests that a target BP of less than 130/80 mmHg is preferable in diabetic patients.

NICE guidance (2002) suggests that first-line antihypertensives should be thiazide diuretics, beta-blockers, ACEIs and ARBs in patients who do not have microalbuminuria.

CCBs should be used as second-line therapy. In patients with microalbuminuria, ACEIs should be used first line as they have a protective effect on the kidney.

4. **What are the recommendations for the management of blood lipids in patients with type 2 diabetes?**
JBS 2 guidelines suggest that statin therapy is recommended for diabetics who are 40 years old or more, and have either type 1 or type 2 diabetes, or for patients with type 1 or type 2 diabetes aged 18–39 and one of the following: retinopathy, nephropathy or poor glycaemic control ($HbA_{1c} > 9\%$), elevated BP requiring antihypertensives, raised cholesterol, features of metabolic syndrome or a family history of premature cardiovascular disease. Targets of treatment are to reach a reduction of total cholesterol by 25% and LDL by 30% or targets of 4 mmol/L or 2 mmol/L respectively, whichever is the greater. NICE guidance stratifies patients according to cholesterol and cardiovascular risk.

5. **When should antiplatelet therapy be initiated in patients with type 2 DM?**
JBS 2 guidelines suggest aspirin for patients with established cardiovascular disease and selected patients with diabetes who are 50 years of age or older, or who are younger but have had the disease for 10 years or more, or who are already receiving treatment for hypertension, once blood pressure has been controlled to <150 mmHg systolic and <90 mmHg diastolic.[b]

6. **Describe the approaches to managing CVD in DM.**
The management of cardiovascular disease is multifactorial and includes smoking cessation, management of dyslipidaemia and hypertension, tight glycaemic control, tackling obesity, and avoiding or reducing any other risk factors.

(Continued)

7. **What are the indications for insulin in type 2 DM?**

Apart from type 1 DM, insulin has a number of indications, including:

- in type 2 DM where patients have inadequate control on oral hypoglycaemic agents
- in type 2 DM where oral hypoglycaemic agents are contraindicated
- impaired glucose tolerance in pregnancy (gestational diabetes mellitus (GDM))
- in patients with type 2 DM who are pregnant
- during the perioperative period, when oral drug-controlled patients are not eating or drinking, and insulin requirements are unstable
- in acute illness in patients with type 2 DM.

Table 2.6

Drug	Mode of action
Biguanides: metformin	• Does not increase pancreatic secretion of insulin (but requires insulin for its action) but rather targets insulin resistance • Decreases glucose output from the liver (gluconeogenesis) • Increases peripheral muscle glucose uptake • Low risk of hypoglycaemia or weight gain: suitable for obese individuals
Sulphonylureas: gliclazide glipizide tolbutamide NB: glibenclamide is long acting and rarely used now	• All produce weight gain (mean 2.8 kg) – use in lean patients • All similarly effective: reduction of HbA$_{1c}$ 1–2% as monotherapy, but after 3 years 50% of patients require combination therapy • Increase insulin secretion by beta-cells and so require residual beta-cell function; risk of hypoglycaemia • Different pharmacokinetic features across class
Glitazones: rosiglitazone pioglitazone	• Reduce insulin resistance; improve sensitivity to insulin in muscle and adipose tissue • May also reduce hepatic glucose output • Rosiglitazone now licensed as triple therapy with metformin and sulphonylurea, but consider alternative – insulin • Increased risk of heart failure
Prandial glucose regulators: repaglinide nateglinide	• Novel hypoglycaemic agents chemically unrelated to sulphonylureas • Require residual beta-cell function; stimulate insulin release via different receptor sites from that of sulphonylureas to target postprandial hyperglycaemia so can be used in patients with non-routine daily patterns • Repaglinide as monotherapy or in combination with metformin, nateglininde only in combination with metformin • Can miss a meal, miss a dose
Alpha-glucosidase inhibitors: acarbose	• Delays the digestion and absorption of starch and sucrose in the small intestine • Taken with the first mouthful of food • Not absorbed so no systemic effects • HbA$_{1c}$ reduction of 0.5–1% • Major limiting factor: flatulence and GI disturbances, so rarely used in practice

→

8. **When is it appropriate to use insulin glargine in type 2 DM?**
   Glargine is not recommended by NICE (2002) for routine use in type 2 DM, but may be considered for patients who require assistance with insulin injections, who have recurrent hypoglycaemia or who would otherwise require twice-daily insulin injections in combination with oral hypoglycaemic agents.

9. **Why is metformin a good choice in type 2 DM?**
   Metformin is a good choice because it does not cause two of the main problems faced by diabetic patients – hypoglycaemia and weight gain. It is thought actually to promote weight loss, possibly because it makes patients feel slightly nauseous and they eat less.

10. **When should glitazones be used in type 2 DM?**
    According to NICE *Technology Appraisal 63* (2003), glitazones should be used as second-line therapy added to metformin or sulphonylureas only when patients are unable to tolerate one of the combination of metformin and a sulphonylurea. In these cases, glitazones should replace the drug that the patient cannot take.

11. **How does each class of oral hypoglycaemic agent act to control blood glucose levels?**
    See Table 2.6.

**Answers to self-assessment questions:
Endocrinology and rheumatology 3:
rheumatoid arthritis** (p. 61)

1. **What are the causes of RA?**
   The causes of RA are uncertain, but it is thought that there are genetic, environmental and infectious triggers of the disease. What is known is that symptoms of disease result from inappropriate inflammatory response caused by cytokines. This leads to a condition that is more than disabling – it is a long-term systemic disease that affects many organ systems throughout the body.

2. **What should be taken into consideration when prescribing NSAIDs?**
   The patient should be assessed for the risk factors for the GI adverse effects of NSAIDs. These include those aged over 65 years, with co-prescription of corticosteroids or anticoagulants or a second NSAID, or with CVD. If an NSAID is needed, try the least potent first, and initiate at, and use, the lowest possible dose. NSAIDs should be taken for the shortest time required by symptoms. Caution should be taken with concomitant ACEIs, lithium and corticosteroids, and in patients with CVD.

3. **What is the role of cyclo-oxygenase 2 (COX-2) inhibitors in the management of RA?**
   Although NICE guidance was published, this may be considered obsolete since the withdrawal of rofecoxib, the only COX-2 thought to have robust data to support a reduction in risk of GI bleeds. There have been a number of different interpretations of the research into COX-2s, and further investigation is required definitively to establish the risks and benefits of COX-2 inhibition over traditional NSAIDs. There are unresolved questions regarding an increase in cardiovascular events, and the co-prescription of COX-2 inhibitors with low-dose aspirin or proton pump inhibitors (PPIs).

(Continued)

4. **At what stage should DMARDs be initiated in RA patients?**

It is now common for patients with newly diagnosed RA to be initiated with DMARD therapy early on in the course of their disease. For many, this is the first step in a management strategy involving increasing or decreasing doses, experiencing side-effects, and for transferring to other, or additional, DMARDs. For some, it will mean taking medicines to counteract or reduce the side-effects of other therapies, and, many years of close monitoring of their biochemical and haematological parameters. While many patients may be used to less noxious drugs such as simple analgesia, the concept of taking potentially toxic medicines may be extremely worrying. For these reasons, the importance of appropriate counselling by the rheumatology team is hugely important.

The use of disease-modifying drugs in rheumatology has become simpler with regard to monotherapy, with most centres using methotrexate or sulfasalazine as first choice. The addition of leflunomide to the DMARD group now means that for the first time in a number of years another effective option exists. There remains a significant amount of debate, however, about what to do next. Although it has become more common to see patients on combinations of DMARDs, early studies suggested that these did not help patients. More recent studies have shown more promise; however, it has been questioned whether these combinations improve outcomes in the longer term.

5. **Why is patient counselling important with DMARDs?**

DMARDs and other medicines used in rheumatology are potentially toxic. In particular, methotrexate has been the subject of a National Patient Safety Agency alert. A number of patients have been harmed as a result of taking or being prescribed methotrexate in an incorrect manner. It is important that they understand that their dose is taken on a weekly and not a daily basis and that they understand that the tablets come in two different strengths: 2.5 mg and 10 mg. See individual DMARD monographs for details in their respective summaries of product characteristics.

6. **What counselling points should be covered in patients receiving DMARDs?**

Patients should be advised that DMARDs may take some time to work (up to 3 months) and that therapy will need to be continued for some time after symptoms have improved to prevent recurrence of disease flares. Patients should be warned that DMARDs may affect their liver, renal or haematological functions or colour body fluids (sulfasalazine), and that they should take precautions with regard to family planning while taking these drugs and for some time afterwards. Patients should also be warned to look for signs of infection and unexplained bruising which may be a sign of drug toxicity, and that blood monitoring is essential.

7. **What advantages does parenteral methotrexate have over oral therapy?**

Although methotrexate is considered by many to be the gold standard DMARD for RA, treatment is often withdrawn due to poor tolerance, particularly GI adverse effects, rather than lack of efficacy. The subcutaneous route is also considered to address any queries over absorption that may have resulted in poor efficacy.

8. **Which biological drugs are available, and what are the differences between them?**

Anti-tumour necrosis factor-α (TNF-α) therapies include infliximab and etanercept which have been available for several years now, and more recently adalimumab has been added to the group. There have been a number of safety concerns, although initial concerns about the incidence of neoplastic disease and general infection have not been quite as prominent as first feared. New concerns about tuberculosis, congestive cardiac failure and demyelinating disorders have since arisen. Although there is a lot of experience with these agents, in 10–15 years' time a clearer picture will exist to establish their safety profile.

There is only one interleukin receptor antagonist therapy, anakinra, which does not appear to have made as great an impact as the TNF-α antagonists. NICE guidance precludes the use of anakinra unless in the context of a clinical trial, or in the situation where patients have been successfully treated with the drug, and stopping therapy would cause a worsening of symptoms. In combination with anti-TNF α therapy, the use of anakinra is not recommended.

9. **What are the differences between the biological therapies in terms of dosing?**
The differences in therapy are listed in Table 2.7. Which drug is to be selected should be put in context with whether patients wish to self-administer or have their drug administered on a weekly basis, or to come into hospital for infusions.

10. **How can pharmacists help RA patients with compliance?**
While it is well known that many patients with RA may have problems opening their medicines, it is somewhat alarming to find that a large proportion of these patients are never offered advice or assistance with this aspect of their treatment. A number of patients have their own ways of dealing with this, such as using a scalpel to cut open foil in blister packaging, but others face a daily struggle to open their medicine containers. Patients with RA often use eye drops to relieve dry eyes, and some products are more suitable, and possibly more effective, than others. MDIs can also be a problem and breath-actuated inhalers are often useful. Again, it is surprising how resourceful some patients are in enabling them to use their own devices.

11. **What options exist for the treatment of neuropathic pain in RA?**
Neuropathic pain can arise due to structural damage around nerves, and can be a serious problem. The drug choices are similar to those used for neuropathic pain in DM. Most commonly tricyclic antidepressants are prescribed as first line, in particular amitriptyline or imipramine. They should be used in doses much lower than those used for depression, for example 10–50 mg at night for neuropathic pain, rather than 100–150 mg at night for depression. Selective serotonin reuptake inhibitors (SSRIs) do not appear to display a similar effect. Antiepileptic drugs are also used to treat neuropathic pain, particularly or more traditionally carbamazepine. Gabapentin has become more commonly prescribed now because it does not have the significant interaction profile of carbamazepine, although it does cause a transient drowsiness which can be minimised by titrating the dose carefully.

(Continued)

Table 2.7

Drug	Nature of drug	Presentation/administration	Dosing schedule
Infliximab (Remicaide)	Chimaeric immunoglobulin G (IgG1) monoclonal antibody	100 mg powder for concentrate for solution for infusion	3 mg/kg given as an IV infusion over a 2 h period, followed by additional 3 mg/kg infusion doses at 2 and 6 weeks after the first infusion, then every 8 weeks thereafter. Dosing is often increased by either increasing the dose per kilogram, and/or reducing the time period between doses. Infliximab must be given concomitantly with methotrexate
Etancercept (Enbrel)	Human tumour necrosis factor receptor p75 Fc fusion protein	50 mg powder and solvent for solution for injection	50 mg reconstituted and administered once weekly as a subcutaneous injection. Based on the TEMPO[a] trial, adding in methotrexate to etanercept improves patient outcomes
Adalimumab (Humira)	Recombinant human monoclonal antibody	40 mg solution for injection in prefilled syringe	40 mg administered every other week as a single dose via subcutaneous injection. Dosing can be increased to a weekly dose if response to therapy is inadequate. Methotrexate should be continued during treatment
Anakinra (Kineret)	Human interleukin 1 receptor antagonist (IL1-RA)	Solution for injection in a prefilled syringe	100 mg daily. NICE suggests that use should only be as part of a clinical trial

[a]Klareskog L, van der Heijde D, de Jager JP, et al. TEMPO (Trial of Etanercept and Methotrexate with Radiographic Patient Outcomes) study investigators. Therapeutic effect of the combination of etanercept and methotrexate compared with each treatment alone in patients with rheumatoid arthritis: double-blind randomized controlled trial. Lancet 2004; 363: 675–681.

N Nephrology and renal transplantation

Introduction

The kidneys are essential for maintaining fluid balance, blood pressure control, organ perfusion and a variety of other homeostatic functions. Impairment may be either acute or chronic, and will affect many other organs. Many elderly patients have a degree of renal impairment, requiring special attention by the pharmacist even though it is often impossible to improve a chronic renal impairment. Fortunately, there is a lot of spare capacity in the kidneys, and much of their function can be lost before it becomes problematic. For the pharmacist, there is an extra consideration. Many drugs (or their metabolites) are excreted in the urine and may accumulate in renal impairment unless there is substantial dose reduction.

 ## Problem 1: the patient has impairment of renal function

The only facts available may be that the serum creatinine is high or urine output has fallen. There are implications for management, prevention of further deterioration in renal function, and drug dose adjustment if normal function is not rapidly restored. A precise diagnosis of the nature and cause of the impairment is essential, although it may be benign, for example after dehydration.

 ## Problem 2: the patient has severe chronic renal disease

Once glomerular filtration rate (GFR) has fallen and remained low, a variety of symptoms present themselves. There comes a point at which dialysis or transplantation will be required to maintain life, usually when the GFR is below 10 mL/min, and often lower, and the patient is said to be in end-stage renal failure (ESRF), although the problems to be dealt with remain the same. Each problem has a small number of specific treatments associated with it, although dietary and fluid management are also important.

 ## Problem 3: the patient has received a renal transplant

About half the 30 000 or so people with ESRF in the UK have a functioning kidney transplant. There is a substantial waiting list due to a shortage of cadaveric (from deceased donors) and live-related (relatives) sources. Following even very successful transplantations, patients may continue to have many of the problems associated with chronic kidney disease in addition to the risks of immunosuppression.

The pharmacist's role

Unfamiliarity makes pharmacists nervous when they come across patients with the problems associated with severe impairment or transplantation. In fact, the management of these conditions is extremely logical, so long as the essential monitoring is carried out and there is an appropriate response to problems. Surprisingly, the major cause of mortality in chronic kidney disease is cardiac disease. Hypertension, fluid overload, uraemia, dislipidaemia, calcium and phosphate problems, and the high prevalence of diabetes all contribute and need to be aggressively addressed. This problem was covered in **Cardiology 4**, although the use of statins and aspirin is not supported by the same evidence base as in CVD patients with no renal impairment, and the drugs themselves may have particular problems in renal disease. Many opportunities exist to empower patients to assist in self-management, build concordance, and improve compliance.

Nephrology and renal transplantation 1 problem: the patient has impairment of renal function

 Objectives of this section

The reader should be able to detail:
- the classification of renal impairment by creatinine clearance
- estimation of creatinine clearance from measurements of serum creatinine
- strategies to delay progression to end-stage renal disease (ESRD)
- consequences of renal failure
- basics of drug dose adjustment in renal impairment
- monitoring required to ensure safety and efficacy of drug therapy.

 Further reading: basics

- *British National Formulary*, current edn. London: Royal Pharmaceutical Society and British Medical Association. Appendix 3: Renal impairment. (ONLINE)

- Morlidge C, Richards T. Managing chronic renal disease. *Pharm J* 2001; 266: 655–658. (ONLINE)
- Sexton JA. Drug use and dosing in the renally impaired adult. *Pharm J* 2003; 271: 231–234. (ONLINE)

 Further reading: moving on

- Walker R, Edwards C, eds. *Clinical Pharmacy and Therapeutics*, 3rd edn. London: Churchill Livingstone; 2003. Chapter 16: Chronic renal failure.
- Dodds LJ, ed. *Drugs in Use*, 3rd edn. London: Pharmaceutical Press; 2003. Chapter 6: Chronic renal failure.

 Guidelines

- Department of Health. *Renal Specific Management of Medicines*. London: Department of Health; 2004. (ONLINE)

 Assessment: renal function estimation

Serum creatinine, a natural breakdown product of muscle turnover, is freely filtered at the glomerulus and so GFR, a good quantitative marker of renal function, is very similar to creatinine clearance (CrCl), and the terms are often used interchangeably (even though they are not quite the same). In addition, unlike most endogenous substances, there is little tubular secretion or reabsorption of creatinine once it has been filtered by the kidney. This means that, as GFR falls, creatinine will rise in a predictable manner, and this makes creatinine the best endogenous reflector of renal function.

CrCl will fall slowly with age, and more rapidly in diabetes and other conditions causing chronic renal failure. Acute deterioration may be secondary to conditions such as dehydration, sepsis, or the initiation of ACEIs/ARBs in a patient with an undiagnosed bilateral renal artery stenosis. CrCl can be calculated from a 24-hour urine collection, though this presents practical difficulties.

Chart 2.11 Nephrology and renal transplantation 1 problem: the patient has impairment of renal function

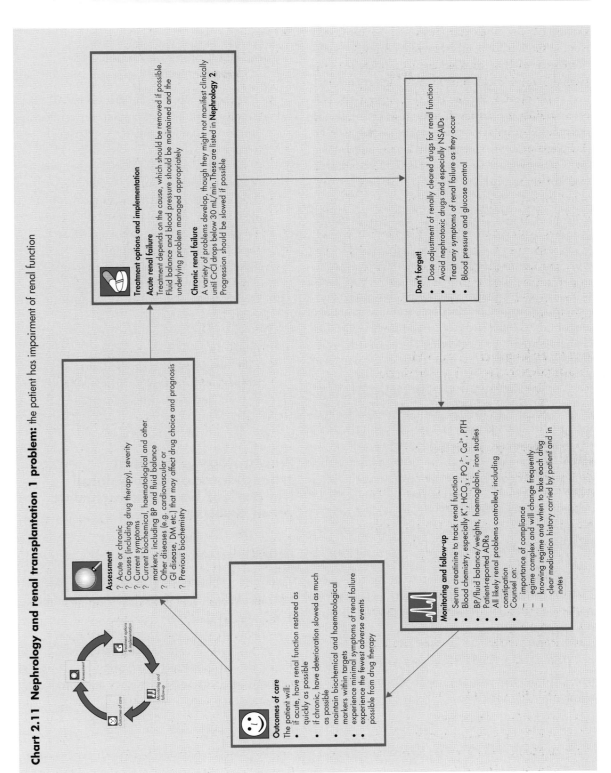

Assessment

? Acute or chronic
? Causes (including drug therapy), severity
? Current symptoms
? Current biochemical, haematological and other markers, including BP and fluid balance
? Other diseases (e.g. cardiovascular or GI disease, DM etc.) that may affect drug choice and prognosis
? Previous biochemistry

Treatment options and implementation

Acute renal failure

Treatment depends on the cause, which should be removed if possible. Fluid balance and blood pressure should be maintained and the underlying problem managed appropriately

Chronic renal failure

A variety of problems develop, though they might not manifest clinically until CrCl drops below 30 mL/min. These are listed in **Nephrology 2**. Progression should be slowed if possible

Don't forget!

- Dose adjustment of renally cleared drugs for renal function
- Avoid nephrotoxic drugs and especially NSAIDs
- Treat any symptoms of renal failure as they occur
- Blood pressure and glucose control

Outcomes of care

The patient will:

- if acute, have renal function restored as quickly as possible
- if chronic, have deterioration slowed as much as possible
- maintain biochemical and haematological markers within targets
- experience minimal symptoms of renal failure
- experience the fewest adverse events possible from drug therapy

Monitoring and follow-up

- Serum creatinine to track renal function
- Blood chemistry, especially K^+, HCO_3^-, PO_4^{3-}, Ca^{2+}, PTH
- BP/fluid balance/weights, haemoglobin, iron studies
- Patient-reported ADRs
- All likely renal problems controlled, including constipation
- Counsel on:
  - importance of compliance
  - regime complex and will change frequently
  - knowing regime and when to take each drug
  - clear medication history carried by patient and in notes

Assessment

Treatment options & implementation

Monitoring and follow-up

Outcomes of care

Creatinine clearance can, however, be estimated from a single serum measurement using an equation such as that of **Cockcroft and Gault**. This (and similar methods in children) relies on the fact that patients of a certain age, weight and sex will produce roughly the same amount of creatinine. If their blood level is x micromoles/L, they will be clearing it at approximately y mL/min, unless their creatinine production is atypical. The equation is well known to pharmacists:

$$CrCl\ (mL/min) = \frac{F \times (140 - \text{age in years}) \times \text{weight (kg)}}{\text{serum creatinine (micromoles/L)}}$$

where $F = 1.04$ (women) and 1.23 (men).

The Cockcroft and Gault equation is valid only in adults, and excludes catabolism and pregnancy (atypical creatinine production), and obesity unless ideal body weight is used. In addition, if CrCl is changing rapidly (e.g. entering or recovering from acute renal failure), serum creatinine may not be changing rapidly enough to reflect this. For example, a creatinine of 400 micromoles/L is high and could either be acutely deranged or chronically high. If the derangement is acute it could be that CrCl has recovered to normal, and time will allow serum creatinine to catch up. Alternatively, the same patient could have a near-zero clearance, and over the next few days serum creatinine will continue to rise further. All changes and derangements in serum creatinine should therefore be investigated and acted on.

The GFR, which in a healthy young adult can be as high as 150 mL/min, declines with age to values of 40 mL/min or less in very elderly people. The *BNF* classifies adult renal function into bands for the purposes of drug dose adjustment, but it will be seen that even mild renal failure may represent the loss of a majority of function. Drug doses may need adjustment, and this is discussed in the self-assessment questions.

SAQ Self-assessment questions:
Nephrology and renal transplantation 1 (Answers on p. 80)

1. If a patient has a serum creatinine on admission of 200 micromoles/L (reference range <110 micromoles/L), what might your impression be?
2. Why bother estimating CrCl rather than simply looking at serum creatinine?
3. What can cause renal function to deteriorate?
4. What should your response be when serum creatinine rises rapidly?
5. Which drug doses need adjusting in the renally impaired patient?
6. Do all drugs with a narrow therapeutic index need reducing?
7. What are the symptoms of renal impairment?
8. Can the progression of renal disease towards ESRF (stage 5 chronic kidney disease) and dialysis be delayed?

Nephrology and renal transplantation 2 problem: the patient has severe chronic renal disease

 Objectives of this section

The reader should be able to detail:
- problems seen as CrCl declines, and the drugs used to manage them
- biochemical and haematological parameters monitored in chronic kidney disease
- drug dosage adjustment in dialysis
- monitoring required for efficacy and safety of drug therapy.

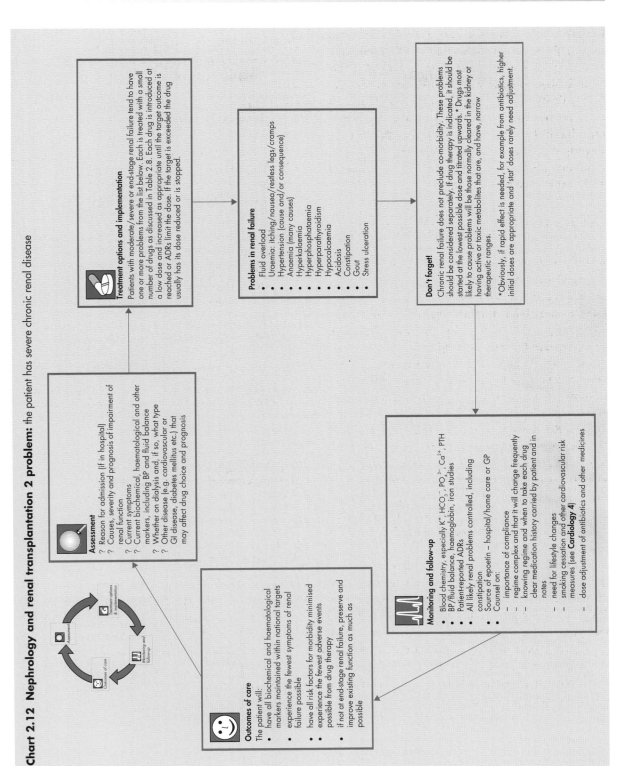

Chart 2.12 Nephrology and renal transplantation 2 problem: the patient has severe chronic renal disease

Assessment
- ? Reason for admission (if in hospital)
- ? Causes, severity and prognosis of impairment of renal function
- ? Current symptoms
- ? Current biochemical, haematological and other markers, including BP and fluid balance
- ? Whether on dialysis and, if so, what type
- ? Other disease (e.g. cardiovascular or GI disease, diabetes mellitus etc.) that may affect drug choice and prognosis

Treatment options and implementation
Patients with moderate/severe or end-stage renal failure tend to have one or more problems from the list below. Each is treated with a small number of drugs as discussed in Table 2.8. Each drug is introduced at a low dose and increased as appropriate until the target outcome is reached or ADRs limit the dose. If the target is exceeded the drug usually has its dose reduced or is stopped.

Problems in renal failure
- Fluid overload
- Uraemia: itching/nausea/restless legs/cramps
- Hypertension (cause and/or consequence)
- Anaemia (many causes)
- Hyperkalaemia
- Hyperphosphataemia
- Hyperparathyroidism
- Hypocalcaemia
- Acidosis
- Constipation
- Gout
- Stress ulceration

Don't forget!
Chronic renal failure does not preclude co-morbidity. These problems should be considered separately. If drug therapy is indicated, it should be started at the lowest possible dose and titrated upwards. * Drugs most likely to cause problems will be those normally cleared in the kidney or having active or toxic metabolites that are, and have, narrow therapeutic ranges.

*Obviously, if rapid effect is needed, for example from antibiotics, higher initial doses are appropriate and 'star' doses rarely need adjustment.

Outcomes of care
The patient will:
- have all biochemical and haematological markers maintained within national targets
- experience the fewest symptoms of renal failure possible
- have all risk factors for morbidity minimised
- experience the fewest adverse events possible from drug therapy
- if not at end-stage renal failure, preserve and improve existing function as much as possible

Monitoring and follow-up
- Blood chemistry, especially K^+, HCO_3^-, PO_4^{3-}, Ca^{2+}, PTH
- BP/fluid balance, haemoglobin, iron studies
- Patient-reported ADRs
- All likely renal problems controlled, including constipation
- Source of epoetin – hospital/home care or GP
- Counsel on:
  - importance of compliance
  - regime complex and that it will change frequently
  - knowing regime and when to take each drug
  - clear medication history carried by patient and in notes
  - need for lifestyle changes
  - smoking cessation and other cardiovascular risk measures (see **Cardiology 4**)
  - dose adjustment of antibiotics and other medicines

Assessment

Treatment options & implementation

Monitoring and follow-up

Outcomes of care

Table 2.8 Some subproblems seen in severe chronic kidney disease

Subproblem	Outcome of treatment	Treatment options and implementation	Monitoring
N2.1: Decline in renal function	GFR will be optimised and preserved as much as possible. This usually involves tight control of blood pressure, protein intake, blood glucose and auto-immune processes. If dialysis becomes necessary (ESRF) function rarely recovers	ACEIs may delay progression of renal failure, especially in patients with diabetes although they are associated with potassium retention	GFR can be calculated from serum creatinine
N2.2: Oligouria	Maximise urine output as much as possible	Loop diuretics used in high doses, often with metolazone	Blood chemistry, fluid balance, weight
N2.3: Uraemia	Low incidence of: itching; nausea; cramps; restless legs	After optimising any dialysis: (a) hydroxyzine/chlorphenamine; (b) metoclopramide/domperidone etc.; (c) quinine salts; (d) clonazepam	Start dose low, increase until symptoms controlled/ adverse events, or maximum dose reached
N2.4: Hypertension	BP to BHS 2004 Standards (see **Cardiology 1**)	All classes except thiazides depending on co-morbidity. Start with low doses and titrated, regardless of hepatic/renal clearance	BP, beware K$^+$ with ACEIs/ARBs, usual ADRs. Reduce doses/withdraw if BP too low or ADRs/may need to withhold before haemodialysis
N2.5: Anaemia	Hb >11 g/dL but not excessive (note: this is a higher European standard)	Ensure iron replete with oral or IV iron, then either epoetin-beta or darbepoetin, subcutaneous (or IV if on high dose). Start low and increase monthly	Hb, BP, iron stores.[a] Increase epoetin/darbepoetin until target Hb obtained; reduce if exceeded
N2.6: Hyperphosphataemia	Serum phosphate <1.78 mmol/L, but also calcium phosphate product <4.4 mmol^2/L^2 as detailed in Renal Association standards and K-DOQI guidelines[b,c]	Control hypocalcaemia, restrict dietary phosphate intake, phosphate binders with meals (calcium carbonate/calcium acetate are usually first-line but aluminium hydroxide may be needed; sevelamer does not add to calcium or aluminium load but is expensive)	Serum PO$_4^{3-}$/Ca^{2+} (adjusted) (Al^{3+} if relevant) Check compliance with diet and timing of doses (with meals). If hypo-phosphataemic, reduce doses. If ADRs, change binder
N2.7: Hypocalcaemia and hyperparathyroidism	Serum calcium in range, calcium phosphate product as described above, PTH no more than 2–3 times upper limit of normal	Alfacalcidol and calcitriol; start low and titrate up	Need to avoid excessive elevation of serum calcium, especially if concurrent calcium-containing phosphate binders
N2.8: Acidosis	Serum bicarbonate in range	Sodium bicarbonate tablets or capsules (more expensive). Start low (600 mg tds) and increase slowly. If on haemodialysis may be able to adjust without oral agents.	Reduce dose if bicarbonate rises too much

Table 2.8 Some subproblems seen in severe chronic kidney disease *(continued)*

Subproblem	Outcome of treatment	Treatment options and implementation	Monitoring
N2.9: Co-prescriptions for other medicines	Patient will receive appropriate dosing of all medicines for degree of renal function.	Consider therapeutic index, whether normally renally cleared or active/ toxic metabolites, start with lower doses	Observe that objectives of therapy, including avoidance of adverse events, are being met
N2.10: Gout	Patient will not experience gout (often aggravated by diuretics)	Allopurinol in reduced doses appropriate for renal function	No attacks; serum urate levels

[a] Sexton JA, Vincent M. Remedying calcium and phosphate problems in chronic kidney disease. *Pharm J* 2004; 274: 561–564. (ONLINE)
[b] Renal Association. *Treatment of Adults and Children with Renal Failure: Standards and audit measures*, 3rd edn. London: Royal College of Physicians of London and the Renal Association; 2002. (ONLINE)
[c] National Kidney Foundation. *Kidney Dialysis Outcomes Quality Initiative (K/DOQI) Clinical Practice Guidelines*. New York: National Kidney Foundation; 2005. (ONLINE)

Further reading: basics

- Morlidge C, Richards T. Managing chronic renal disease. *Pharm J* 2001; 266: 655–658 (ONLINE)
- Currie A, O'Brien P. Renal replacement therapies. *Pharm J* 2001; 266: 675–679. (ONLINE)

Further reading: moving on

- Sexton JA, Vincent M. Managing anaemia in renal failure. *Pharm J* 2004; 273: 603–605. (ONLINE)
- Sexton JA, Vincent M. Remedying calcium and phosphate problems in chronic kidney disease. *Pharm J* 2004; 274: 561–564. (ONLINE)
- Walker R, Edwards C, eds. *Clinical Pharmacy and Therapeutics*, 3rd edn. London: Churchill Livingstone; 2003. Chapter 16: Chronic renal failure.
- Dodds LJ, ed. *Drugs in Use*, 3rd edn. London: Pharmaceutical Press; 2003. Chapter 6: Chronic renal failure.

Guidelines

- Renal Association. *Treatment of Adults and Children with Renal Failure: Standards and audit measures*, 3rd edn. London: Royal College of Physicians of London and the Renal Association; 2002. (ONLINE)
- National Kidney Foundation. *Kidney Dialysis Outcomes Quality Initiative (K/DOQI) Clinical Practice Guidelines*. New York: National Kidney Foundation; 2005. (ONLINE)

SAQ Self-assessment questions:
Nephrology and renal transplantation 2 (Answers on p. 82)

1. What effect does dialysis have on drug dosing?
2. A patient is still anaemic while receiving weekly subcutaneous darbepoetin 30 micrograms. Should the dose be increased?
3. Should calcium carbonate be prescribed for hypocalcaemia in chronic kidney disease?
4. A patient has a normal serum calcium and yet the doctor has increased the alfacalcidol/calcitriol dose. Why?
5. Which treatment is best for hypertension in severe renal impairment?

Nephrology and renal transplantation 3 problem: the patient has received a renal transplant

Objectives of this section

The reader should be able to detail:

- the use of immunosuppression to prevent rejection
- selection of an appropriate immunosuppression regime
- monitoring required to optimise graft and patient survival and health
- complications of long-term therapy and counselling required by patients.

Further reading: basics

- *British National Formulary*, current edn. London: Royal Pharmaceutical Society and British Medical Association. Section 8.2: Drugs affecting the immune response. (ONLINE)
- Lee M, Devaney A. Immunosuppression after adult renal transplant. *Pharm J* 2001; 266: 789–791. (ONLINE)

Further reading: moving on

- Walker R, Edwards C, eds. *Clinical Pharmacy and Therapeutics*, 3rd edn. London: Churchill Livingstone; 2003. Chapter 16: Chronic renal failure.
- Dodds LJ, ed. *Drugs in Use*, 3rd edn. London: Pharmaceutical Press; 2003. Chapter 7: Renal transplantation.

Guidelines

- National Institute for Clinical Excellence. *Technology Appraisal 85: The Clinical Effectiveness and Cost Effectiveness of Immuno-suppressive Therapy for Renal Transplantation*. London: NICE; 2004.

SAQ Self-assessment questions:
Nephrology and renal transplantation 3 (Answers on p. 83)

1. How can the optimal prognosis of a new kidney be ensured?
2. What initial immunosuppression regime is the best?
3. What are the big dangers of immunosuppression?
4. What are the adverse effects of the specific drugs?
5. What is chronic rejection?
6. Are there non-nephrotoxic immunosuppressants that could be used as the primary anti-rejection therapy?
7. After transplantation, can all other 'renal' drugs be stopped?
8. What should be the approach to the admission to hospital of a patient who has received a transplant that is working well?
9. What other pharmaceutical points are important in the care of a transplant recipient?

Chart 2.13 Nephrology and renal transplantation 3 problem: the patient has received a renal transplant

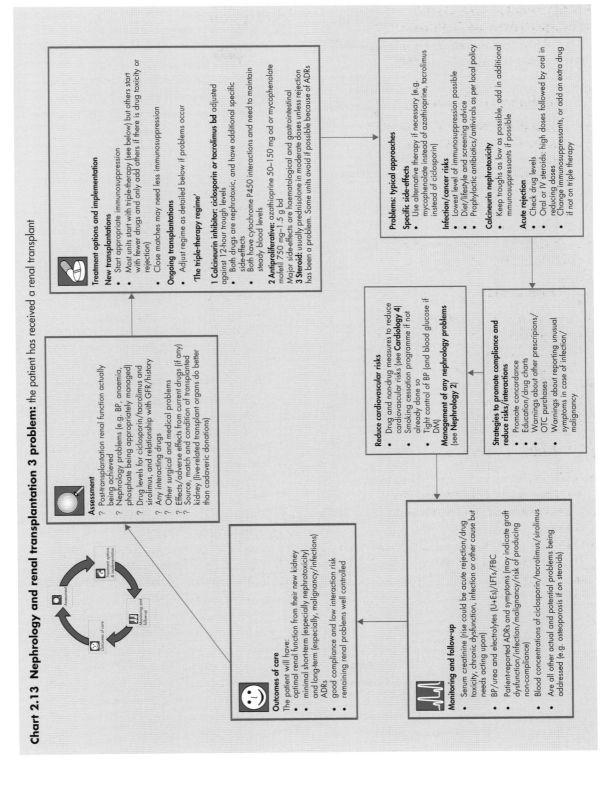

Assessment

? Post-transplantation renal function actually being achieved
? Nephrology problems (e.g. BP, anaemia, phosphate being appropriately managed)
? Drug levels for ciclosporin/tacrolimus and sirolimus, and relationship with GFR/history
? Any interacting drugs
? Other surgical and medical problems
? Effects/adverse effects from current drugs (if any)
? Source, match and condition of transplanted kidney (live-related transplant organs do better than cadaveric donations)

Treatment options and implementation

New transplantations
- Start appropriate immunosuppression
- Most units start with triple-therapy (see below) but others start with fewer drugs and only add others if there is drug toxicity or rejection)
- Close matches may need less immunosuppression

Ongoing transplantations
- Adjust regime as detailed below if problems occur

'The triple-therapy regime'

1 **Calcineurin inhibitor: ciclosporin or tacrolimus bd** adjusted against 12-hour trough levels
- Both drugs are nephrotoxic, and have additional specific side-effects
- Both have cytochrome P450 interactions and need to maintain steady blood levels

2 **Antiproliferative:** azathioprine 50–150 mg od or mycophenolate mofetil 750 mg–1.5 g bd
Major side-effects are haematological and gastrointestinal

3 **Steroid:** usually prednisolone in moderate doses unless rejection has been a problem. Some units avoid if possible because of ADRs

Problems: typical approaches

Specific side-effects
- Use alternative therapy if necessary (e.g. mycophenolate instead of azathioprine, tacrolimus instead of ciclosporin)

Infection/cancer risks
- Lowest level of immunosuppression possible
- Diet/lifestyle and screening advice
- Prophylactic antibiotics/antivirals as per local policy

Calcineurin nephrotoxicity
- Keep troughs as low as possible, add in additional immunosuppressants if possible

Acute rejection
- Check drug levels
- Oral or IV steroids: high doses followed by oral in reducing doses
- Change immunosuppressants, or add an extra drug if not on triple therapy

Reduce cardiovascular risks
- Drug and non-drug measures to reduce cardiovascular risks (see **Cardiology 4**)
- Smoking cessation programme if not already done so
- Tight control of BP (and blood glucose if DM)

Management of any nephrology problems (see **Nephrology 2**)

Strategies to promote compliance and reduce risks/interactions
- Promote concordance
- Education/drug charts
- Warnings about other prescriptions/ OTC purchases
- Warnings about reporting unusual symptoms in case of infection/ malignancy

Monitoring and follow-up
- Serum creatinine (rise could be acute rejection/drug toxicity, chronic dysfunction, infection or other cause but needs acting upon)
- BP/urea and electrolytes (U+Es)/LFTs/FBC
- Patient-reported ADRs and symptoms (may indicate graft dysfunction/infection/malignancy/risk of producing non-compliance)
- Blood concentrations of ciclosporin/tacrolimus/sirolimus
- Are all other actual and potential problems being addressed (e.g. osteoporosis if on steroids)

Outcomes of care
The patient will have:
- optimal renal function from their new kidney
- minimal short-term (especially nephrotoxicity) and long-term (especially, malignancy/infections) ADRs
- good compliance and low interaction risk
- remaining renal problems well controlled

Answers to self-assessment questions:
Nephrology and renal transplantation 1: impairment of renal function (p. 74)

1. **If a patient has a serum creatinine on admission/appointment of 200 micromoles/L (reference range <110 micromoles/L), what would your impression be?**
Application of Cockcroft and Gault's estimation to this patient suggests that their CrCl is in the order of 30–60 mL/min, depending on sex, age and weight. For example, if the patient were a man of 60 years of age and 70 kg, the maths would look like this:

$$CrCl = \frac{1.23 \times (140 - 60) \times 70}{200} = about\ 34\ mL/min$$

In a younger patient, this is unusual, and two possibilities are evident. The patient may genuinely have *BNF* mild or borderline renal impairment, in which case the question must be 'why?'. Remember that the method of Cockcroft and Gault cannot be applied if the patient is catabolic, pregnant, and so forth, when there may be abnormal creatinine production. Alternatively either the patient may have dehydration and you are seeing a contribution from concentration, or they are in acute renal failure due to sepsis, hypotension, hypovolaemia, a new ACEI or one of many other causes. In these cases it is difficult to determine whether their acute renal failure is worsening, and creatinine will continue to rise, or whether it is recovering and creatinine is falling again. In acute situations, causative factors should be controlled or removed, infection treated, hydration maintained and serum creatinine rechecked 12–24 hours later.

2. **Why bother estimating CrCl rather than simply looking at serum creatinine?**

Serum creatinine alone does not enable an objective assessment of renal function. For example, elderly patients may be in mild renal failure, but simply because of their lower muscle mass and turnover have a serum creatinine in the reference range. As mentioned, a single measurement of serum creatinine will not respond quickly to changes in CrCl, and without a previous result a raised figure cannot differentiate an acute from a chronic deterioration. However, a raised serum creatinine is a useful marker that all might not be well in the kidneys. In addition, using the method of Cockcroft and Gault, it can provide a surprisingly accurate estimate of CrCl in the stable patient.

3. **What can cause renal function to deteriorate?**
GFR declines with age until death, but is usually sufficient to provide no symptoms even in old age. However, deterioration will be accelerated in patients with elevated blood pressure, diabetes mellitus and many other conditions. Sometimes no single cause can be found. Tight control of blood pressure and blood glucose, and the introduction of ACEIs may slow the progression of renal failure in many patients.

4. **What should your response be when serum creatinine rises rapidly?**
A rapidly rising serum creatinine usually reflects an acute deterioration in renal function. This is common in conditions such as shock, sepsis and dehydration, all causes of 'prerenal' failure. It can also reflect outflow obstructions in the kidney or ureters and these are examples of 'postrenal' causes of renal failure. If the cause is corrected quickly enough, renal function can often be rapidly restored. Various auto-immune conditions can cause renal

→

failure and these are usually treated with powerful immunosuppressants and high-dose steroids.

Drugs can also cause renal failure. Many drugs are nephrotoxic by a variety of routes but acute failure is commonly implicated with the introduction of ACEIs in the presence of an undiagnosed bilateral renal artery stenosis. Overzealous administration of diuretics can deplete the central compartment and renal perfusion, and NSAIDs can suppress renal prostaglandins which help maintain renal blood flow. Renal prostaglandins are especially important where there is a pre-existing renal impairment, including that seen in elderly people.

5. **Which drug doses need adjusting in the renally impaired patient?**

Few drugs need any reduction at all until the GFR falls below 50 mL/min. The drugs which need adjusting are those that are renally cleared (or those that have any renally cleared metabolites, which are either biologically active or toxic). In addition, the therapeutic index needs to be considered. An example of this is given for two common renally cleared antibiotics in Table 2.9. The typical dose reductions needed in renal failure are shown for amoxicillin (wide therapeutic window) and ceftazidime (narrow therapeutic window).

All company summaries of product characteristics (SPCs) and the *BNF* provide extra information. Drugs that are renally cleared, and have a narrow therapeutic window, and are also nephrotoxic present particular problems. A good example of this is gentamicin and this should be used with extreme caution in renally impaired patients.

6. **Do all drugs with a narrow therapeutic index need reducing?**

Just as it was shown above that not all renally cleared drugs need a dose reduction, so not all drugs with a narrow therapeutic index need a dose reduction either. Phenytoin, carbamazepine and theophylline are all examples of drugs where tight control of blood levels is essential, but no dose reduction in renal impairment is needed. This is because they are all completely metabolised in the liver, with no active metabolites.

7. **What are the symptoms of renal impairment?**

In the early stages, none at all. Many patients present with moderate-to-severe renal failure, months away from needing dialysis, having had no problems for most of the course of their deterioration, which may have been progressing silently over many years. Eventually patients may present with oedema or breathlessness,

Table 2.9 Dose reductions of amoxicillin and ceftazidime recommended in renal failure

GFR	Classification	Amoxicillin	Ceftazidime
>50 mL/min	Normal	500 mg tds	1 g tds
20–50 mL/min	Mild renal impairment	500 mg tds	1 g bd
10–20 mL/min	Moderate renal impairment	500 mg tds	1 g od
<10 mL/min	Severe renal impairment	250 mg tds	1 g alternate days

(Continued)

hypertension, anaemia, tiredness and so forth, due to the build-up of fluid and toxins. These symptoms may not present until the GFR has fallen to 20–30 mL/min, and 75% of normal function has already been lost.

8. **Can the progression towards ESRF (stage 5 chronic kidney disease) and dialysis be delayed?**
If a causative factor can be identified and controlled, there may be benefits. For instance, the tight control of blood pressure and glucose in type 2 diabetes, combined with the use of ACEIs, may delay progression. Steroids may be of considerable benefit in auto-immune kidney disease. However, in many patients, the progression of kidney disease is unrelenting and the date at which dialysis will be needed can be predicted months in advance by considering the rate of decline of the GFR.

 Answers to self-assessment questions: Nephrology and renal transplantation 2: severe chronic renal disease (p. 77)

1. **What effect does dialysis have on drug dosing?**
Most of the treatments associated with chronic kidney disease are titrated against a measurable response: so long as dosing is initiated gently and the response monitored there should be no need to consider the degree of renal impairment or whether dialysis has been initiated. This applies to drugs such as the following, doses of which tend to be constantly adjusted:
- sodium bicarbonate (bicarbonate)
- darbepoetin/epoetin (haemoglobin)
- IV and oral iron (ferritin and transferrin saturation)
- phosphate binders (phosphate)
- alfacalcidol/calcitriol (serum calcium/PTH)
- antihypertensive drugs (BP).

Other medicines become problematic usually only if they (or their active metabolites) have a large proportion of renal clearance and a narrow therapeutic window. Drugs that are removed by peritoneal dialysis or haemodialysis tend to be those that are renally cleared normally. Continuous ambulatory peritoneal dialysis tends to mimic severe renal failure and haemodialysis has short periods of high clearance followed by long periods of negligible clearance. This can be a problem if a drug is given once daily – digoxin and gentamicin are given after the haemodialysis session has finished.

2. **A patient is still anaemic while receiving weekly subcutaneous darbepoetin 30 micrograms. Should the dose be increased?**
What is the serum haemoglobin? It is not usual to treat anaemia until the normal reference range for an individual is achieved. This is expensive and may increase risks of complications. The current European guidelines are satisfied if haemoglobin is >11 g/dL. How long have they been taking the darbepoetin for? It may simply be that it has not had long enough to work? At least a month is needed to judge effect. Has the patient got a minor active bleed? The most important question to ask if all the above are resolved is about the availability of iron to fuel erythropoiesis, as measured by transferrin saturation and serum ferritin. Finally infection and uncontrolled uraemia, hyperparathyroidism and

$\rightarrow$

hyperaluminiumaemia can all diminish response. If all the above are controlled, doses of darbepoetin can be increased by 25% at a time, continuing to monitor response and blood pressure.

3. **Should calcium carbonate be prescribed for hypocalcaemia in chronic kidney disease?**
Not usually – it is prescribed to bind dietary phosphate and prevent phosphate absorption. Calcium levels are brought up by the administration of activated vitamin D sterols. However, this is an oversimplification and the most recent US guidelines do express concern about calcium loads, and their effects on serum calcium and calcium phosphate product, which is associated with soft-tissue calcification.

Vitamin D precursors made in the skin or taken in the diet or in supplements, such as pharmaceuticals containing ergocalciferol or colecalciferol, are of no use in renal disease. The kidney is responsible for their hydroxylation to active vitamin D and so, if it cannot perform this function, alfacalcidol (1-alpha-hydroxycolecalciferol) or calcitriol (1,25-dihydroxycolecalciferol) is needed instead to maintain calcium levels.

4. **A patient has a normal serum calcium and yet the doctor has increased the alfacalcidol/calcitriol dose. Why?**
Almost certainly because the PTH is elevated, and another indication for these drugs is to suppress the secondary hyperparathyroidism that develops in renal failure. However, the ability to suppress PTH is limited by the calcium-raising effect that vitamin D will have. This can be reduced by 'pulsing' the vitamin D, giving it only on 2–3 days each week.

5. **Which treatment is best for hypertension in severe renal impairment?**
All classes except thiazides (which are ineffective when the GFR is low) can be used depending on other co-morbidities. ACEIs and ARBs are more likely to cause hyperkalaemia, which prevents dose optimisation or use in many patients. The need to use three or four drugs from all classes is frequently observed, and less usual treatments such as the alpha-blocker doxazosin are frequently employed as options run out.

Answers to self-assessment questions:
Nephrology and renal transplantation 3: renal transplant
(p. 78)

1. **How can the optimal prognosis of a new kidney be ensured?**
The donor and recipients need compatible blood groups. In addition, the closest possible cellular (human leucocyte antigen (HLA)) tissue typing match should be ensured between the donor kidney and the recipient. This is one of the current assignment conditions of the scarce cadaveric kidneys made available in the UK.

The recipient should have been exposed to as few foreign human antigens as possible, usually from blood transfusions or previous transplantations. Finally, kidneys should be placed with caution into patients who have shown poor compliance with drug therapy, diet or dialysis while awaiting transplantation.

2. **What initial immunosuppression regime is the best?**
There is no proven answer to this. The most common regime in the UK involves either ciclosporin or tacrolimus in combination with mycophenolate mofetil and

(Continued)

prednisolone, the so-called triple-therapy regime. Some units prefer ciclosporin, others tacrolimus. Other units start with ciclosporin as monotherapy and add other drugs if needed. There is no good evidence to say which approach generates the most surviving kidneys and patients at, say, 10 years post-transplantation.

3. **What are the big dangers of immunosuppression?**

It would be possible to prevent virtually all acute rejection with heavy immunosuppression, but this would come with an unacceptably high risk of the two most important adverse events in the long term. The first of these is infection, and patients are counselled to avoid certain raw foods and have good hygiene. There is also a risk of unusual infections such as *Pneumocystis carinii* pneumonia (PCP) or cytomegalovirus, especially in newly transplanted patients. (Some, but not all, units routinely give prophylactic antibiotics and antivirals for three months after transplantation.) Secondly, there is a higher risk of malignant diseases, both solid tumours and a variety of lymphomas. The lightest possible immunosuppression is therefore preferable, and units that 'go in heavy' will reduce doses and withdraw drugs over time.

4. **What are the adverse effects of the specific drugs?**

Steroids cause their own problems – weight gain, diabetes and bone problems – and azathioprine and mycophenolate have a reputation for GI disturbances. The real problem with the calcineurin inhibitors, ciclosporin and tacrolimus, is that they are extremely nephrotoxic. If levels are too high then the kidney can be forced into acute renal failure, but even at apparently normal blood levels there is some damage occurring. Ciclosporin and tacrolimus also have their own peculiar adverse effect profiles as can be seen in the *BNF*.

5. **What is chronic rejection?**

Most transplant staff now talk about 'chronic graft dysfunction', which is the ongoing decline in the CrCl of the transplanted kidney over time, as opposed to the 'acute rejection' seen in the new transplant when the chosen regime is inadequate to prevent an acute renal failure from occurring. The reason that 'chronic rejection' is a fading term is that the reasons for graft decline are probably multifactoral, involving rejection processes, drug toxicity, infections, hypertension and other factors. It is managed by keeping the patient under regular review and adjusting the immunosuppression regime to respond to rises in serum creatinine.

6. **Are there non-nephrotoxic immunosuppressants that could be used as the primary anti-rejection therapy?**

Sirolimus is the only currently licensed drug available in the UK to belong to this new generation of therapies. It is licensed for use in combination with ciclosporin and steroids for the first three months after transplantation, after which the ciclosporin is withdrawn. Some units are using sirolimus but others prefer to wait for more long-term evidence about efficacy and safety to emerge.

7. **After transplantation, can all other 'renal' drugs be stopped?**

Some kidneys work excellently after transplantation for many years, while others struggle along at just above the level of function that would necessitate a return to dialysis. Regardless of graft function, every

$\rightarrow$

patient should be treated as an individual. Some will still need sodium bicarbonate, phosphate binders, alfacalcidol and erythropoietic therapies, adjusted against response in the usual manner (see **Nephrology 2**).

8. **What should be the approach to the admission to hospital of a patient who has received a transplant that is working well?**
Pharmacists should ensure that the regime that the patient is on is maintained, and that interacting therapies are avoided unless essential (and then with monitoring of blood levels). If renal function deteriorates, the transplant unit or nearest nephrologists should be consulted for advice.

9. **What other pharmaceutical points are important in the care of a transplant recipient?**
Compliance should be promoted, and the avoidance of OTC therapies such as NSAIDs or St John's wort that might affect renal function or interact with the immunosuppression regime. Ciclosporin, tacrolimus and sirolimus have narrow therapeutic windows and careful monitoring of levels and the avoidance of interacting drugs are important. Cardiac risks are the biggest problem and lifestyle advice, low-dose aspirin, statins and antihypertensives should be used as appropriate (see **Cardiology 4**).

G Gastroenterology

Chapter contents

Introduction

Problems involving the GI system are commonly encountered in primary care and are responsible for a significant number of hospital admissions. Four major problems encountered are listed below.

Problem 1: the patient has upper gastrointestinal disease

Both peptic ulcer disease (PUD) and gastro-oesophageal reflux disease (GORD) fall into this category. Significant causes of gastric and duodenal ulceration include administration of NSAID drugs (including low-dose aspirin) and *Helicobacter pylori* infection. Diagnosis is confirmed by endoscopy and if untreated can result in complications such as bleeding. GORD ranges from minor indigestion and heartburn to recurrent episodes which can result in oesophagitis (diagnosed with endoscopy).

Problem 2: the patient has inflammatory bowel disease

Inflammatory bowel disease (IBD) encompasses ulcerative colitis (UC) and Crohn's disease (CD). Both diseases are chronic relapsing–remitting conditions which may require hospitalisation during severe exacerbations. Although advances in treatments have been made, a number of patients will eventually require surgery. Patients with Crohn's disease may have numerous surgical resections over the years which can impact on their nutritional status as well as drug absorption.

Problem 3: the patient is an abuser of alcohol

Patients may drink excess quantities of alcohol for a variety of reasons including depression or as a social habit. Chronic alcohol abuse is associated with a variety of health problems including liver cirrhosis and heart disease. Patients with a high alcohol intake who suddenly stop drinking are at risk of alcohol withdrawal, a syndrome that can range from mild agitation to a life-threatening condition that includes seizures and coma.

Problem 4: the patient has chronic liver disease

There are numerous factors that can cause chronic liver disease, alcohol consumption being the most common. Chronic liver disease results in a number of symptoms that require treatment, and carries a significant mortality. In addition drug choice and dosing may be affected if the patient has liver disease.

The pharmacist's role

Patients with upper GI symptoms often visit their community pharmacist before consulting their GP. The community pharmacist will be able to recommend advice and treatment to patients with mild upper or lower GI symptoms, but has a responsibility to refer any patient presenting with persistent or 'alarm' symptoms (e.g. weight loss, dysphagia) to their GP. Patients with IBD are often prescribed immunosuppressant therapy which requires detailed counselling and stringent monitoring. The pharmacist has an important role in advising on the choice and dosing of drugs in patients with liver disease.

Gastroenterology 1 problem: the patient has upper gastrointestinal disease

 Objectives of this section

The reader should be able to detail:
- the objectives of care for patients presenting with PUD and GORD
- the contributory factors to the above conditions
- the treatment options available:
  PUD:
  — proton pump inhibitors (PPIs)
  — H_2-receptor antagonists
  GORD:
  — antacids and alginates
  — H_2-receptor antagonists
  — PPIs
- monitoring required to ensure efficacy and safety of drug therapy.

 Further reading: basics

- *British National Formulary*, current edn. London: Royal Pharmaceutical Society and British Medical Association. Section 1.1:

Dyspepsia and gastro-oesophageal reflux disease. (ONLINE)
- Randall MD, Neil KE. *Disease Management*. London: Pharmaceutical Press; 2004. Chapter 7: Dyspepsia and peptic ulcer disease.
- Walker R, Edwards C, eds. *Clinical Pharmacy and Therapeutics*, 3rd edn. London: Churchill Livingstone; 2003. Chapter 10: Peptic ulcer disease.
- Dodds LJ, ed. *Drugs in Use*, 3rd edn. London: Pharmaceutical Press; 2003. Chapter 8: Duodenal ulcer.

 Further reading: moving on

- Harris A, Misiewicz JJ. ABC of the upper gastrointestinal tract: management of *Helicobacter pylori* infection. *BMJ* 2001; 323: 1047–1050. (ONLINE)
- de Caestecker J. ABC of the upper gastrointestinal tract: oesophagus: heartburn. *BMJ* 2001; 323: 736–739. (ONLINE)
- Veysey M, Wilkinson M. Today's management of dyspepsia and ulcers. *Prescriber* 2003; 14: 52–62. (ONLINE)

 Guidelines

- National Institute for Clinical Excellence. *Clinical Guideline 17: Dyspepsia: Managing dyspesia in adults in primary care*. London: NICE; 2004.

 Self-assessment questions: Gastroenterology 1 (Answers on p. 96)

1. How do NSAIDs (and low-dose aspirin) cause gastric and duodenal ulcers?
2. What factors need to be considered when choosing a regime for the eradication of *H. pylori*?
3. What counselling points should be discussed with a patient prescribed a regime for eradication of *H. pylori*?

(Questions continued on page 89)

Chart 2.14 Gastroenterology 1 problem: the patient has upper gastrointestinal disease

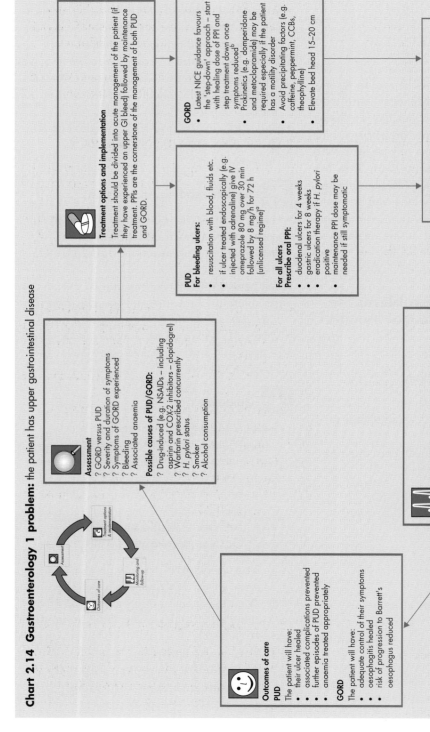

Assessment

? GORD versus PUD
? Severity and duration of symptoms
? Symptoms of GORD experienced
? Bleeding
? Associated anaemia

Possible causes of PUD/GORD:

? Drug-induced (e.g. NSAIDs – including aspirin and COX2 inhibitors – clopidogrel)
? Warfarin prescribed concurrently
? H. pylori status
? Smoker
? Alcohol consumption

Treatment options and implementation

Treatment should be divided into acute management of the patient (if they have experienced an upper GI bleed) followed by maintenance treatment. PPIs are the cornerstone of the management of both PUD and GORD.

PUD
For bleeding ulcers:

- resuscitation with blood, fluids etc.
- if ulcer treated endoscopically (e.g. injected with adrenaline) give IV omeprazole 80 mg over 30 min followed by 8 mg/h for 72 h (unlicensed regime)[a]

For all ulcers
Prescribe oral PPI:

- duodenal ulcers for 4 weeks
- gastric ulcers for 8 weeks
- eradication therapy if H. pylori positive
- maintenance PPI dose may be needed if still symptomatic

GORD

- Latest NICE guidance favours the 'step-down' approach – start with healing dose of PPI and step treatment down once symptoms reduced[b]
- Prokinetics (e.g. domperidone and metoclopramide) may be required especially if the patient has a motility disorder
- Avoid precipitating factors (e.g. caffeine, peppermint, CCBs, theophylline)
- Elevate bed head 15–20 cm

Don't forget!

If the patient was admitted to hospital as a result of their symptoms and was taking aspirin, clopidogrel, NSAID, COX-2 inhibitors, warfarin, complete a yellow card and send to the CSM. Even if the drug is not black triangle the ADR still needs to be reported if it results in or prolongs hospitalisation. The following information will be required:

- suspected drugs along with doses and date they were started
- details of reaction including OGD report
- treatment given including blood transfusion
- blood tests – Hb, urea (raised during an upper GI bleed), creatinine – on admission and at least one further set of results

Monitoring and follow-up
PUD

- Monitor for symptoms associated with ulcer, e.g. abdominal pain, indigestion
- Patients with gastric ulcers or complicated duodenal ulcers will require repeat endoscopy to ensure that ulcer has healed
- H. pylori status will be rechecked to ensure eradication
- Check Hb and iron studies

GORD

- Monitor symptomatic control
- Symptomatic control correlates with healing of oesophagitis

Outcomes of care
PUD

The patient will have:

- their ulcer healed
- associated complications prevented
- further episodes of PUD prevented
- anaemia treated appropriately

GORD

The patient will have:

- adequate control of their symptoms
- oesophagitis healed
- risk of progression to Barrett's oesophagus reduced

[a]Lau JYW, Sung JJY, Lee KKC et al. Effect of intravenous omeprazole on recurrent bleeding after endoscopic treatment of bleeding peptic ulcers. N Engl J Med 2000; 343: 310–315.
[b]National Institute for Clinical Excellence. Clinical Guideline 17. Dyspepsia: Managing dyspepsia in adults in primary care. London: NICE; 2004. (ONLINE)

**Self-assessment questions:
Gastroenterology 1** (Continued)

4. A patient who has received omeprazole 20 mg od for 4 weeks after an endoscopy has revealed that they have a duodenal ulcer. What treatment should the patient receive after this?
5. List the major factors that can predispose a patient to GORD.
6. What is meant by the 'step-up' and 'step-down' approaches for the management of GORD?

Gastroenterology 2 problem: the patient has inflammatory bowel disease

 Objectives of this section

The reader should be able to detail:
- the objectives of care in patients with IBD
- the difference between ulcerative colitis and Crohn's disease
- **the management UC:**
  — steroids
  — 5-aminosalicylates (5-ASAs)
  — azathioprine/mercaptopurine
- **the management of CD:**
  — dietary therapy
  — steroids
  — 5-ASAs
  — azathioprine/mercaptopurine
  — methotrexate
  — antibiotics
  — infliximab
- monitoring required to ensure efficacy and safety of drug therapy.

 Further reading: basics

- *British National Formulary*, current edn. London: Royal Pharmaceutical Society and British Medical Association. Section 1.5: Chronic bowel disorders. (ONLINE)
- Walker R, Edwards C, eds. *Clinical Pharmacy and Therapeutics*, 3rd edn. London: Churchill Livingstone; 2003. Chapter 11: Inflammatory bowel disease.
- Dodds LJ, ed. *Drugs in Use*, 3rd edn. London: Pharmaceutical Press; 2003. Chapter 9: Ulcerative colitis.

 Further reading: moving on

- Rampton DS. Regular review: management of Crohn's disease. *BMJ* 1999; 319: 1480–1485. (ONLINE)
- Ghosh S, Shand A, Ferguson A. Regular review: ulcerative colitis. *BMJ* 2000; 320: 1119–1123. (ONLINE)

 Guidelines

- Carter MJ, Lobo AJ, Travis SPL. Guidelines for the management of inflammatory bowel disease in adults. *Gut* 2004; 53 (Suppl V): v1–v16. (ONLINE)
- Scott EM, Gaywood I, Scott BB. Guidelines for osteoporosis in coeliac disease and inflammatory bowel disease. *Gut* 2000; 46 (Suppl I): I1–I18. (ONLINE)
- National Institute for Clinical Excellence. *Technology Appraisal 40: The Clinical Effectiveness and Cost Effectiveness of Infliximab for Crohn's Disease*. London: NICE; 2002. (ONLINE)

 **Self-assessment questions:
Gastroenterology 2** (Answers on p. 97)

1. List four differences between UC and CD.
2. Why should corticosteroids be avoided in the long-term management of IBD?

(Questions continued on page 91)

Chart 2.15 Gastroenterology 2 problem: the patient has inflammatory bowel disease

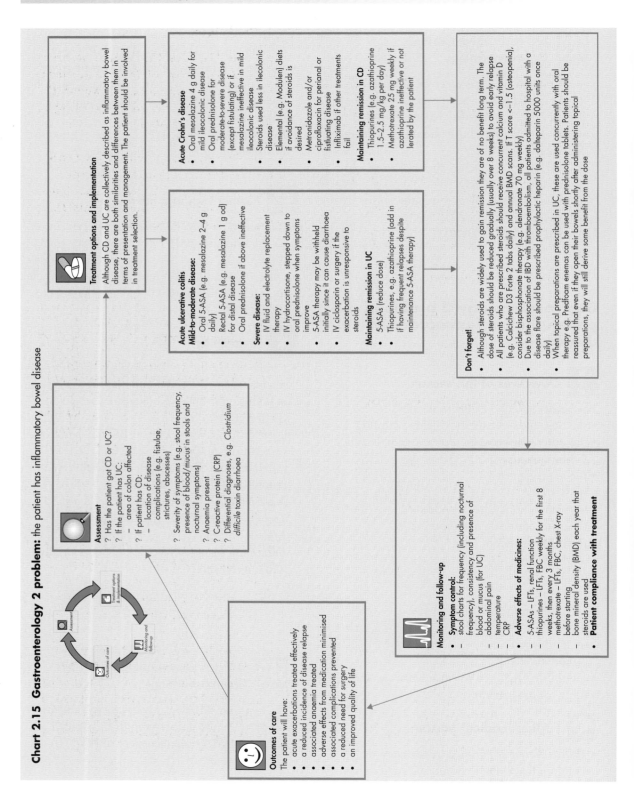

Assessment

? Has the patient got CD or UC?
? If the patient has UC:
  – area of colon affected
? If patient has CD:
  – location of disease
  – complications (e.g. fistulae, strictures, abscesses)
? Severity of symptoms (e.g. stool frequency, presence of blood/mucus in stools and nocturnal symptoms)
? Anaemia present
? C-reactive protein (CRP)
? Differential diagnoses, e.g. *Clostridium difficile* toxin diarrhoea

Treatment options and implementation

Although CD and UC are collectively described as inflammatory bowel disease, there are both similarities and differences between them in terms of presentation and management. The patient should be involved in treatment selection.

Acute ulcerative colitis
Mild-to-moderate disease:
- Oral 5-ASA (e.g. mesalazine 2–4 g daily)
- Rectal 5-ASA (e.g. mesalazine 1 g od) for distal disease
- Oral prednisolone if above ineffective

Severe disease:
- IV fluid and electrolyte replacement therapy
- IV hydrocortisone, stepped down to oral prednisolone when symptoms improve
- 5-ASA therapy may be withheld initially since it can cause diarrhoea
- IV ciclosporin or surgery if the exacerbation is unresponsive to steroids

Maintaining remission in UC
- 5-ASAs (reduce dose)
- Thiopurines, e.g. azathioprine (add in if having frequent relapses despite maintenance 5-ASA therapy)

Acute Crohn's disease
- Oral mesalazine 4 g daily for mild ileocolonic disease
- Oral prednisolone for moderate-to-severe disease (except fistulating) or if mesalazine ineffective in mild ileocolonic disease
- Steroids used less in ileocolonic disease
- Elemental (e.g. Modulen) diets if avoidance of steroids is desired
- Metronidazole and/or ciprofloxacin for perianal or fistulating disease
- Infliximab if other treatments fail

Maintaining remission in CD
- Thiopurines (e.g. azathioprine 1.5–2.5 mg/kg per day)
- Methotrexate 25 mg weekly if azathioprine ineffective or not tolerated by the patient

Don't forget!
- Although steroids are widely used to gain remission they are of no benefit long term. The dose of steroids should be reduced gradually (usually over 8 weeks) to avoid early relapse
- All patients who are prescribed steroids should receive concurrent calcium and vitamin D (e.g. Calcichew D3 Forte 2 tabs daily) and annual BMD scans. If T score <–1.5 (osteopenia), consider bisphosphonate therapy (e.g. alendronate 70 mg weekly)
- Due to the association of IBD with thromboembolism, all patients admitted to hospital with a disease flare should be prescribed prophylactic heparin (e.g. dalteparin 5000 units once daily)
- When topical preparations are prescribed in UC, these are used concurrently with oral therapy e.g. Predfoam enemas can be used with prednisolone tablets. Patients should be reassured that even if they open their bowels shortly after administering topical preparations, they will still derive some benefit from the dose

Monitoring and follow-up
- **Symptom control:**
  – stool charts for frequency (including nocturnal frequency), consistency and presence of blood or mucus (for UC)
  – abdominal pain
  – temperature
  – CRP
- **Adverse effects of medicines:**
  – 5-ASAs – LFTs, renal function
  – thiopurines – LFTs, FBC weekly for the first 8 weeks, then every 3 months
  – methotrexate – LFTs, FBC, chest X-ray before starting
  – bone mineral density (BMD) each year that steroids are used
- **Patient compliance with treatment**

Outcomes of care

The patient will have:
- acute exacerbations treated effectively
- a reduced incidence of disease relapse
- associated anaemia treated
- adverse effects from medication minimised
- associated complications prevented
- a reduced need for surgery
- an improved quality of life

SAQ Self-assessment questions:
Gastroenterology 2 (Continued)

3. Why are 5-ASAs not used for all patients with IBD?
4. Describe the role of immunosuppressants in IBD.
5. A patient with UC is having repeated exacerbations despite treatment with balsalazide. What additional treatment options are available?
6. What is the role of infliximab in IBD?
7. Which groups of drugs should be avoided or used with caution in a patient with IBD?
8. Why might patients with IBD also suffer from anaemia?
9. Why may intravenous iron infusions be required by some patients with CD?

Gastroenterology 3 problem: the patient is an abuser of alcohol

 Objectives of this section

The reader should be able to detail:
- the symptoms associated with alcohol withdrawal
- the treatment of acute alcohol withdrawal
- the complications associated with vitamin deficiencies that people with alcohol problems are at risk of developing
- monitoring required to ensure efficacy and safety of drug therapy.

 Further reading: basics

- Mason P. Alcohol misuse – a case study. *Pharm J* 2003; 271: 777–779. (ONLINE)
- Dodds LJ, ed. *Drugs in Use*, 3rd edn. London: Pharmaceutical Press; 2003. Chapter 10: Alcoholic liver disease.

 Guidelines

- Thompson AD, Cook CH, Touquet R, Henry JA. The Royal College of Physicians report on alcohol: guidelines for managing Wernicke's encephalopathy in the accident and emergency department. *Alcohol Alcohol* 2002; 37: 513–521. (ONLINE)
- Scottish Intercollegiate Guidelines Network. *SIGN 74: The Management of Harmful Drinking and Alcohol Dependence in Primary Care: A national clinical guideline* (2003). Edinburgh: SIGN. (ONLINE)

SAQ Self-assessment questions:
Gastroenterology 3 (Answers on p. 99)

1. What are the maximum recommended weekly limits of alcohol intake for men and women?
2. A patient is transferred to your ward for treatment of acute alcohol withdrawal. Why is it important to administer treatment to this patient?
3. A common starting dose of chlordiazepoxide is 20 mg qds. For how long should this treatment be continued?
4. If the patient were jaundiced, would chlordiazepoxide be an appropriate treatment?
5. Describe the monitoring that is required for a patient receiving chlordiazepoxide therapy.
6. The patient asks you why they have been prescribed thiamine and multivitamin tablets since they don't like taking tablets. How would you deal with this question?
7. What other treatment should be considered in this group of patients?

Chart 2.16 Gastroenterology 3 problem: the patient is an abuser of alcohol

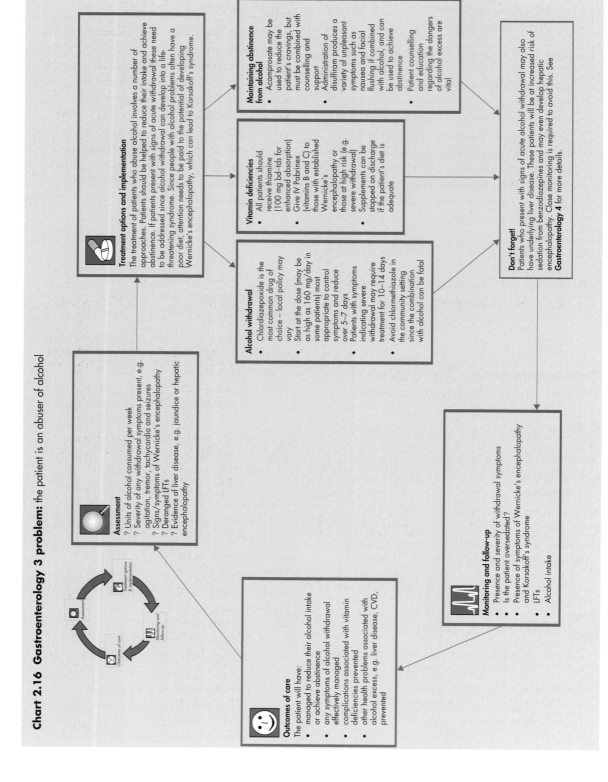

Treatment options and implementation

The treatment of patients who abuse alcohol involves a number of approaches. Patients should be helped to reduce their intake and achieve abstinence. If patients present with signs of acute withdrawal these need to be addressed since alcohol withdrawal can develop into a life-threatening syndrome. Since people with alcohol problems often have a poor diet, attention needs to be paid to the potential of developing Wernicke's encephalopathy, which can lead to Korsakoff's syndrome.

Maintaining abstinence from alcohol

- Acamprosate may be used to reduce the patient's cravings, but must be combined with counselling and support
- Administration of disulfiram produces a variety of unpleasant symptoms such as nausea and facial flushing if combined with alcohol, and can be used to achieve abstinence
- Patient counselling and education regarding the dangers of alcohol excess are vital

Vitamin deficiencies

- All patients should receive thiamine (100 mg bd-tds for enhanced absorption)
- Give IV Pabrinex (vitamins B and C) to those with established Wernicke's encephalopathy or those at high risk (e.g. severe withdrawal)
- Supplements can be stopped on discharge if the patient's diet is adequate

Alcohol withdrawal

- Chlordiazepoxide is the most common drug of choice – local policy may vary
- Start at the dose (may be as high as 160 mg/day in some patients) most appropriate to control symptoms and reduce over 5–7 days
- Patients with symptoms indicating severe withdrawal may require treatment for 10–14 days
- Avoid chlormethiazole in the community setting since the combination with alcohol can be fatal

Don't forget!

Patients who present with signs of acute alcohol withdrawal may also have underlying liver disease. These patients will be at increased risk of sedation from benzodiazepines and may even develop hepatic encephalopathy. Close monitoring is required to avoid this. See **Gastroenterology 4** for more details.

Assessment

- ? Units of alcohol consumed per week
- ? Severity of any withdrawal symptoms present, e.g. agitation, tremor, tachycardia and seizures
- ? Signs/symptoms of Wernicke's encephalopathy
- ? Deranged LFTs
- ? Evidence of liver disease, e.g. jaundice or hepatic encephalopathy

Monitoring and follow-up

- Presence and severity of withdrawal symptoms
- Is the patient oversedated?
- Presence of symptoms of Wernicke's encephalopathy and Korsakoff's syndrome
- LFTs
- Alcohol intake

Outcomes of care

The patient will have:
- managed to reduce their alcohol intake or achieve abstinence
- any symptoms of alcohol withdrawal effectively managed
- complications associated with vitamin deficiencies prevented
- other health problems associated with alcohol excess, e.g. liver disease, CVD, prevented

Assessment

Treatment options & implementation

Monitoring and follow-up

Outcomes of care

Gastroenterology 4: the patient has chronic liver disease

Objectives of this section

The reader should be able to detail:

- the objectives of care in patients with chronic liver disease
- the common problems in chronic liver disease and how they may be treated
  — ascites – spironolactone, loop diuretics

— hepatic encephalopathy – lactulose, enemas, metronidazole, neomycin
— portal hypertension (and varices) – propranolol
— pruritis associated with jaundice – colestyramine, topical applications
— coagulopathy – vitamin K
- the effects of altered drug handling in liver disease
- monitoring required to ensure efficacy and safety of drug therapy.

Table 2.10 Some subproblems seen in chronic liver disease

Subproblem	Outcome of treatment	Assessment and implementation	Treatment options	Monitoring
G4.1: Jaundice	• Relieve itching • Reduce bilirubin levels	• Cholestasis or hepatitis? • Presence of pruritis	• Colestyramine 4 g bd • Oral antihistamines less effective • Consider topical preparations such as calamine lotion or menthol 1% in aqueous cream	• Bilirubin level • Symptom control
G4.2: Coagulopathy (raised prothrombin time)	• Avoid bleeds • Correct as best as possible	• Cholestasis or cirrhosis • Prothrombin time (or INR)	• Vitamin K IV for 3 days in cirrhosis • Use oral menadiol in cholestasis/obstruction • Avoid NSAIDs	• Prothrombin time • Signs of bleeding
G4.3: Hypoalbuminaemia	• Avoid problems from low albumin	• Albumin level • Implications for other problems	• Diet • Routine albumin infusions not used unless other problems present	• Albumin level
G4.4: Ascites	• Remove fluid/prevent reaccumulation • Avoid electrolyte disturbances • Avoid renal impairment	• Precipitating factors • Severity • Presence of spontaneous bacterial peritonitis (SBP)	• Fluid restriction and salt-free diet • Spironolactone 100–400 mg/day • Frusemide 40–160 mg daily if peripheral oedema or spironolactone alone ineffective • Paracentesis (drain) in refractory ascites	• Daily weight – aim to lose maximum 1 kg/day • Fluid balance • U+Es twice weekly

(Continued on page 94)

Table 2.10 Some subproblems seen in chronic liver disease *(continued)*

Subproblem	Outcome of treatment 😊	Assessment and implementation 🔍	Treatment options	Monitoring
G4.5: Hepatic encephalopathy	• Prevent progression • Reverse	• Precipitating factors, e.g. sedatives, infection, constipation, electrolyte disturbances (e.g. low Na⁺), GI bleeds • Grade by severity	• Remove/treat precipitating factors • Lactulose: up to 40 mL tds • Enemas if still not opening bowels • Neomycin in resistant cases	• Symptoms and consciousness level • Stool frequency: aim for two to three loose stools per day without diarrhoea
G4.6: portal hypertension	• Reduce portal pressure • Avoid/heal varices • Avoid variceal bleeds	Presence of varices on endoscopy	• Propranolol 20–40 mg bd • Isosorbide mononitrate used less often due to possibility of increased mortality associated with its use in these patients	• Pulse: aim for 25% reduction or resting pulse of 60 beats/min • BP
G4.7: Altered drug handling	• Avoid drug-related problems	• Severity of disease (Child–Pugh score) • Drugs prescribed	• Lower the dose of hepatically cleared drugs • Use renally cleared drugs instead	• Response to therapy • Plasma concentration if applicable

Further reading: basics

- *British National Formulary*, current edn. London: Royal Pharmaceutical Society and British Medical Association. Appendix 2: Liver disease. (ONLINE)
- Walker R, Edwards C, eds. *Clinical Pharmacy and Therapeutics*, 3rd edn. London: Churchill Livingstone; 2003. Chapter 14: Liver disease.
- Randall MD, Neil KE. *Disease Management*. London: Pharmaceutical Press; 2004. Chapter 10: The liver patient.

Further reading: moving on

- Kennedy PT, O'Grady JG. Diseases of the liver: chronic liver disease. *Hosp Pharm* 2002; 9: 137–143. (ONLINE)
- Kriege JEJ, Beckingham IJ. ABC of diseases of liver, pancreas, and biliary system. Portal hypertension – 1: varices. *BMJ* 2001; 322: 348–351. (ONLINE)
- Kriege JEJ, Beckingham IJ. ABC of diseases of liver, pancreas, and biliary system. Portal hypertension – 2: ascites, encephalopathy, and other conditions. *BMJ* 2001; 322: 416–418. (ONLINE)

Chart 2.17 Gastroenterology 4 problem: the patient has chronic liver disease

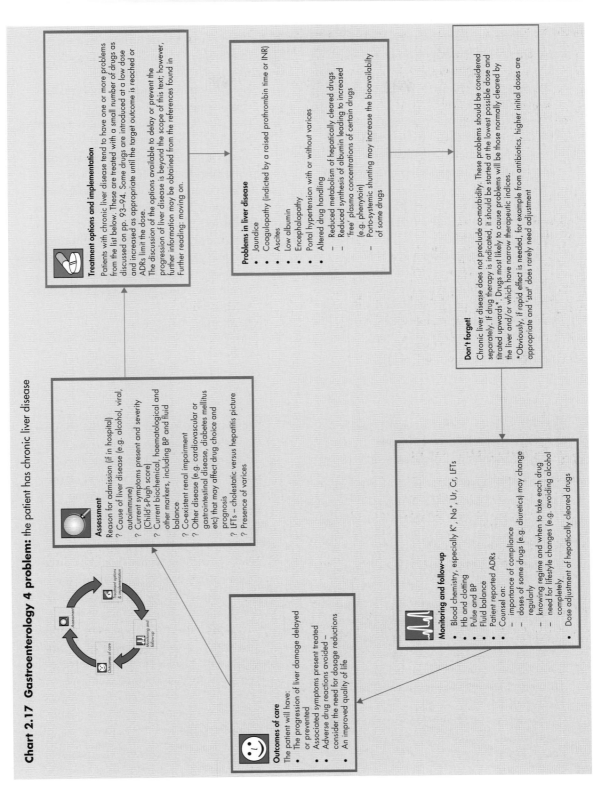

Treatment options and implementation

Patients with chronic liver disease tend to have one or more problems from the list below. These are treated with a small number of drugs as discussed on pp. 93–94. Some drugs are introduced at a low dose and increased as appropriate until the target outcome is reached or ADRs limit the dose.

The discussion of the options available to delay or prevent the progression of liver disease is beyond the scope of this text; however, further information may be obtained from the references found in Further reading; moving on.

Problems in liver disease

- Jaundice
- Coagulopathy (indicated by a raised prothrombin time or INR)
- Ascites
- Low albumin
- Encephalopathy
- Portal hypertension with or without varices
- Altered drug handling
  - Reduced metabolism of hepatically cleared drugs
  - Reduced synthesis of albumin leading to increased 'free' plasma concentrations of certain drugs (e.g. phenytoin)
  - Porto-systemic shunting may increase the bioavailability of some drugs

Don't forget!

Chronic liver disease does not preclude co-morbidity. These problems should be considered separately. If drug therapy is indicated, it should be started at the lowest possible dose and titrated upwards*. Drugs most likely to cause problems will be those normally cleared by the liver and/or which have narrow therapeutic indices.

*Obviously, if rapid effect is needed, for example from antibiotics, higher initial doses are appropriate and 'stat' does rarely need adjustment

Assessment

Reason for admission (if in hospital)
- ? Cause of liver disease (e.g. alcohol, viral, autoimmune)
- ? Current symptoms present and severity (Child's-Pugh score)
- ? Current biochemical, haematological and other markers, including BP and fluid balance
- ? Co-existent renal impairment
- ? Other disease (e.g. cardiovascular or gastrointestinal disease, diabetes mellitus etc) that may affect drug choice and prognosis
- ? LFTs – cholestatic versus hepatitis picture
- ? Presence of varices

Monitoring and follow-up

- Blood chemistry, especially K⁺, Na⁺, Ur, Cr, LFTs
- Hb and clotting
- Pulse and BP
- Fluid balance
- Patient reported ADRs
- Counsel on:
  - importance of compliance
  - doses of some drugs (e.g. diuretics) may change regularly
  - knowing regime and when to take each drug
  - need for lifestyle changes (e.g. avoiding alcohol completely
- Dose adjustment of hepatically cleared drugs

Outcomes of care

The patient will have:
- The progression of liver damage delayed or prevented
- Associated symptoms present treated
- Adverse drug reactions avoided – consider the need for dosage reductions
- An improved quality of life

Self-assessment questions:
Gastroenterology 4 (Answers on p. 100)

1. What is the difference between hepatitis and cirrhosis?
2. When faced with interpreting a patient's LFTs, it is often useful to determine if the patient has a cholestatic picture or hepatitis. How is this determined from a patient's LFTs?
3. Why is vitamin K required by some patients with liver disease, and which forms should be given to them?
4. Describe the four mechanisms that contribute to the treatment of ascites.
5. Discuss the options available to treat ascites.
6. How does hepatic encephalopathy develop and how should it be managed?

7. What is the role of neomycin in the treatment of hepatic encephalopathy?
8. Briefly describe how hepatic encephalopathy differs from Wernicke's encephalopathy.
9. Describe the pharmacological treatment of bleeding oesophageal varices. Why are GI bleeds especially worrying in a patient with liver disease?
10. Which groups of drugs should be used cautiously in a patient with liver disease and why?
11. Which drug would be the best option for the management of the following problems in a patient with liver disease:
    - pain associated with a sprained ankle?
    - depression?
    - epilepsy?

Answers to self-assessment questions:
Gastroenterology 1: upper gastrointestinal disease (p. 87)

1. **How do NSAIDs (and low-dose aspirin) cause gastric and duodenal ulcers?**
   Acidic NSAIDs have a direct irritant effect on the GI mucosa. NSAIDs exert their systemic effects by inhibiting the COX enzymes, which are responsible for the production of prostaglandins. By blocking a COX-1 enzyme, NSAIDs inhibit the production of the physiological prostaglandins which have a protective role. Prostaglandin protects the GI mucosa by increasing bicarbonate and mucus production, stimulating epithelial cell proliferation and regulating basal acid secretion.
2. **What factors need to be considered when choosing a regime for the eradication of H. pylori?**

The main factors that need to be considered are: local resistance patterns to the antibiotics used, patient sensitivity to antibiotics, alcohol consumption (avoid metronidazole if unlikely to abstain from alcohol) and formulary choice of PPI. Examples of licensed eradication regimes can be found in the *BNF*.

3. **What counselling points should be discussed with a patient prescribed a regime for eradication of H. pylori?**
   The patient needs to be counselled on:
   - **the reason for medication** – the purpose of the regime is to kill bacteria in the gut and reduce the chances of ulcer recurrence
   - **the dose and duration of medicines** – all medicines are twice daily for a week, acid suppressor then reduced to once daily and continued for 4–8 weeks to heal the ulcer

$\rightarrow$

- **the importance of compliance** – need to complete the course, missed doses greatly reduce the efficacy of the regime and can result in recurrence of PUD
- **adverse effects** – main side-effects are nausea, vomiting and diarrhoea
- **additional precautions** – avoid alcohol if prescribed metronidazole as it can result in a syndrome that includes severe nausea and facial flushing.

4. **A patient has received omeprazole 20 mg od for 4 weeks after an endoscopy revealed that they have a duodenal ulcer. What treatment should the patient receive after this?**

If the patient remains asymptomatic, then no further treatment is required. Persistent symptoms may indicate that another condition (e.g. GORD) may be responsible for their symptoms and this should be treated accordingly. Recurrent cases of ulceration would require long-term treatment with a PPI. If the patient's ulcer had been due to NSAID use and they required a NSAID (for example, in severe RA), it would be necessary to restart the PPI with the NSAID to prevent ulceration.

5. **List the major factors that can predispose a patient to GORD.**

Drugs (e.g. nitrates, CCBs, theophylline) can lower the gastro-oesophageal sphincter tone and predispose the patient to reflux symptoms. Some foodstuffs (e.g. caffeine, spicy food and peppermint) and pregnancy can also lower the gastro-oesophageal sphincter tone. Patients with motility disorders are also at risk of GORD since delayed emptying of the gastric contents is more likely to result in reflux of the contents.

6. **What is meant by the 'step-up' and 'step-down' approaches for the management of GORD?**

The 'step-up' approach involves starting with antacid and stepping up to H_2-receptor antagonist then a PPI depending on the severity of symptoms.

The 'step-down' approach involves starting with PPI and stepping down to H_2 antagonist then an antacid once symptoms have been controlled.

Current NICE guidance favours the 'step-down' approach.

 Answers to self-assessment questions: Gastroenterology 2: inflammatory bowel disease (p. 89)

1. **List four differences between UC and CD**
See Table 2.11.

2. **Why should corticosteroids be avoided in the long-term management of IBD?**
There is no evidence to support the use of corticosteroids for the maintenance of remission of IBD. They do not heal fistulae, abscesses or ulceration associated with the disease. In addition, long-term steroids are associated with numerous adverse effects: osteoporosis, diabetes, hypertension and Cushing's syndrome.

3. **Why are 5-ASAs not used for all patients with IBD?**
There is less evidence for using 5-ASAs in CD than there is for UC, although they are more effective in purely colonic CD. In UC they should be the cornerstone of long-term management: their use has been shown to reduce the risk of colon cancer in these patients.

4. **Describe the role of immunosuppressants in IBD.**
- UC: ciclosporin has been shown to be effective in severe flares that are steroid resistant (unlicensed use). Azathioprine is used to help maintain remission in

(Continued)

Table 2.11 Differences between ulcerative colitis and Crohn's disease

Ulcerative colitis	Crohn's disease
Affects large intestine only	Can affect any part of the GI tract from the lips to the anus
Inflammation is continuous and superficial	Inflammation is patchy ('skip lesions' may exist) and transmural (affects the full thickness of the bowel)
Smoking may help the disease	Smoking has an adverse effect on the disease
Surgery presents a cure for the disease	Surgery does not cure the disease – it may return to another part of the GI tract
Fistulae and abscesses not associated with the disease	Complications such as abscesses and fistulae may occur

patients who are not effectively managed on a 5-ASA product.

- **CD**: azathioprine is the main therapy used to maintain remission.

All immunosuppressants require monitoring of FBC, LFTs (ciclosporin also requires monitoring of renal function; serum creatinine should not rise by more than a third during ciclosporin therapy).

5. **A patient with UC is having repeated exacerbations despite treatment with balsalazide. What additional treatment options are available?**

Azathioprine (1.5–2.5 mg/kg per day) could be added to try to reduce exacerbations and maintain disease remission. If this approach was unsuccessful or the patient was not keen to take this drug, then surgery should be considered.

6. **What is the role of infliximab in IBD?**

Infliximab is licensed for use in CD where other treatments have failed. NICE guidance recommends that it be used in acute disease that has failed to respond to conventional treatment (e.g. steroids, immunosuppressants or antibiotics). Infliximab is now licensed for the management of severe active UC in patients who have had an inadequate response to conventional therapy.

7. **Which groups of drugs should be avoided or used with caution in a patient with IBD?**

Opioids and anticholinergics should be avoided in acute colitis due to the risk of bowel dilatation and toxic megacolon (which can result in bowel perforation). The use of NSAIDs should be avoided if possible since they may precipitate disease flares. The oral contraceptive pill should be used with caution due to the risk of thromboembolism (patients with IBD are at increased risk of thromboembolism).

8. **Why might patients with IBD also suffer from anaemia?**

UC patients often experience bloody diarrhoea during acute attacks and may lose blood as a result of this.

Crohn's patients may not absorb sufficient quantities of iron and may receive inadequate iron from the diet if the disease affects their appetite. Patients whose disease affects the terminal ileum may also suffer from vitamin B_{12} deficiency anaemia, since this vitamin is absorbed at the terminal ileum. These patients will often require vitamin B_{12} injections every 3 months.

9. **Why may intravenous iron infusions be required by some patients with CD?**

Anaemia is associated with CD. Oral iron preparations have GI side-effects (e.g. nausea, diarrhoea and constipation) which may exacerbate a patient's disease symptoms. If patients cannot tolerate a particular preparation of oral iron, they should be tried on another. If the second preparation cannot be tolerated, intravenous iron may be required.

Answers to self-assessment questions:
Gastroenterology 3: alcohol abuse
(p. 91)

1. **What are the maximum recommended weekly limits of alcohol intake for men and women?**
The maximum recommended alcohol intake for men is 21 units per week and for women it is 14 units per week. A unit of alcohol represents half a pint of 'ordinary' strength beer or lager (i.e. not premium lager), one pub measure of spirits or one glass of wine.

2. **A patient is transferred to your ward for treatment of acute alcohol withdrawal. Why is it important to administer treatment to this patient?**
Acute alcohol withdrawal, if left untreated, can result in minor agitation or develop into a life-threatening syndrome which includes seizures and coma.

3. **A common starting dose of chlordiazepoxide is 20 mg qds. For how long should this treatment be continued?**
Treatment should be reviewed daily and reduced to zero (to avoid dependence) over a period of 5–7 days in most patients. However, it should be noted that some patients suffer with severe withdrawal symptoms and may require up to 14 days' treatment. Some practitioners advocate using a set reducing regime (with daily monitoring of the patient), whereas others adjust the dose on a daily basis. There is no agreement regarding which set regime should be used; variation exists between hospital trusts. In addition to the regular doses of chlordiazepoxide prescribed, patients may also require 'prn' doses to treat breakthrough of withdrawal symptoms.

4. **If the patient were jaundiced, would chlordiazepoxide be an appropriate treatment?**
Jaundice can be an indicator of liver disease. Chlordiazepoxide is a benzodiazepine, which may accumulate in patients with liver disease and precipitate hepatic encephalopathy. Oxazepam is the preferred benzodiazepine in patients with liver disease since it has a shorter half-life and is less likely to accumulate. However, it is not 100% safe in patients with liver disease, so patients should be monitored closely and the lowest dose possible used to control symptoms.

5. **Describe the monitoring that is required for a patient receiving chlordiazepoxide therapy.**
The patient should be assessed on a daily basis for signs of alcohol withdrawal (e.g. tremor, agitation, pulse rate). They should also be monitored to ensure that they are not over-sedated (or developing hepatic encephalopathy) on the current dose of chlordiazepoxide.

6. **The patient asks you why they have been prescribed thiamine and multivitamin tablets since they don't like taking tablets. How would you deal with this question?**
Explain that patients who drink excessive quantities of alcohol are at risk of vitamin deficiencies due to poor diet and reduced absorption of vitamin B. A deficiency of thiamine is particularly worrying since they may develop Wernicke's encephalopathy, which can develop into Korsakoff's syndrome where patients have difficulty in acquiring new memories. They should be reassured that if their diet improves, these tablets may be stopped.

(Continued)

7. **What other treatment should be considered in this group of patients?**
These patients should be offered support and advice to help them stop drinking alcohol in order to avoid complications associated with alcohol abuse, e.g. liver disease, weight gain, ischaemic heart disease and heart failure. In some groups of patients acamprosate may be considered to help them abstain from alcohol; however, since the studies combined this with counselling, it is unclear which component had the most significant effect.

 Answers to self-assessment questions: Gastroenterology 4: chronic liver disease (p. 96)

1. **What is the difference between hepatitis and cirrhosis?**
Hepatitis is a term used to describe inflammation of the liver; it is not just associated with viruses. This is usually seen in acute disease and can be reversed if the underlying cause is treated/removed.

   Cirrhosis is caused by the liver becoming fibrous in nature as a result of continued assault of alcohol, viruses, autoantibodies etc. This form of damage to the liver is irreversible.

2. **When faced with interpreting a patient's LFTs, it is often useful to determine if the patient has a cholestatic picture or hepatitis. How is this determined from a patient's LFTs?**
Since hepatitis describes inflammation of the liver, the patient's serum transaminases (e.g. alanine transaminase (ALT)) will be raised, indicating acute injury. The patient's bilirubin may also be raised, but their alkaline phosphatase (ALP) and gamma-glutamyl transferase (GGT) may be normal or only marginally raised.

   Cholestatis may result from obstruction of the biliary tree. In addition to having a raised bilirubin, these patients will have a raised ALP (and sometimes a raised GGT), but their ALT will be normal or only marginally raised.

3. **Why is vitamin K required by some patients with liver disease, and which forms should be given to them?**
Vitamin K (phytomenadione) is a fat-soluble vitamin required for the production of certain clotting factors. Patients with cholestatic liver disease have problems absorbing oral fat-soluble vitamins. Menadiol is a water-soluble form of vitamin K and may be given to these patients. Alternatively IV vitamin K (phytomenadione) may be used since this overcomes any worries regarding absorption.

   Patients with cirrhosis of the liver may also have clotting abnormalities. However, administration of vitamin K is less effective in these patients since their liver is so badly damaged that they are unable to utilise the vitamin K to produce clotting factors.

4. **Describe the four mechanisms that contribute to the treatment of ascites.**
   - Portal hypertension drives fluid into the peritoneum.
   - Reduced aldosterone metabolism by the liver results in salt and water retention.
   - Reduced albumin synthesis by the liver, results in reduced plasma oncotic

pressure. Thus, fluid leaks out of the circulation into the tissues.

- The renin–angiotensin–aldosterone system is activated due to central depletion (although patients with ascites are fluid overloaded; the fluid is in the wrong compartment).

5. **Discuss the options available to treat ascites.**
Spironolactone (an aldosterone antagonist) is the drug of choice. Start at 100 mg daily and increase by 100 mg every 3–4 days until a maximum of 400 mg daily is reached. You will need to monitor U+Es, fluid balance, daily weights (aim to lose 0.5–1 kg per day).

Loop diuretics may be added if spironolacone alone is not effective or if the patient also has peripheral oedema, e.g. frusemide 40–160 mg daily.

In addition, patients should be put on a salt-free diet and be fluid restricted. (1–1.5 L/day).

In resistant cases the ascites may be drained using paracentesis. These patients must also receive albumin infusions (100 ml of 20% albumin for every 2–3 L drained), to avoid movement of fluid from the central compartment back into the peritoneum.

6. **How does hepatic encephalopathy develop and how should it be managed?**
The liver is responsible for metabolising nitrogenous waste. If damaged it is less efficient at this and these compounds accumulate. Nitrogenous compounds are toxic to the brain, and high levels can result in hepatic encephalopathy which ranges from agitation and mild sedation to severe drowsiness and even coma. The condition may be precipitated by a variety of factors including: sedative drugs, constipating drugs, infection, electrolyte disturbances (especially sodium), major upper GI bleed (increasing the nitrogen load in the gut) and worsening liver disease.

Treatment involves removing any possible precipitating factors and ensuring that the patient is opening the bowels regularly. Lactulose reduces the transit time of bowel contents and reduces bowel pH (thus reducing reabsorption of nitrogenous waste and bacterial growth). The dose used is higher than that for constipation and is titrated to ensure that the patient is producing two to three soft stools per day without experiencing diarrhoea.

7. **What is the role of neomycin in the treatment of hepatic encephalopathy?**
Bacteria are believed to be responsible for the production of nitrogenous waste. Neomycin is an antibiotic with a level of absorption from the gut that is insignificant in most patients. It reduces the bacterial load in the gut and thus reduces the production of nitrogenous waste. Neomycin is reserved for patients who fail to respond to lactulose due to concerns over safety, especially in renal impairment, since it is both nephrotoxic and ototoxic if it accumulates.

8. **Briefly describe how hepatic encephalopathy differs from Wernicke's encephalopathy.**
Wernicke's encephalopathy develops as a result of thiamine deficiency and can develop in patients who do not have liver disease. Hepatic encephalopathy develops only in patients who have liver disease. The symptoms also differ – sedation is unlikely in Wernicke's encephalopathy. The treatments for the two conditions are also different – see earlier questions.

9. **Describe the pharmacological treatment of bleeding oesophageal varices. Why are GI bleeds especially worrying in a patient with liver disease?**
The initial treatment involves blood transfusions and IV fluids to restore the

(Continued)

circulating volume. Vasopressin analogues (e.g. terlipressin) reduce splanchnic blood flow and are used to stop bleeding. Intravenous vitamin K may be given if the patient's INR is raised.

Propranolol (a non-selective beta-blocker) is used to lower the portal pressure and prevent rebleeding.

GI bleeds are particularly worrying in patients with liver disease due to their impaired coagulation.

10. **Which groups of drugs should be used cautiously in a patient with liver disease and why?**

NSAIDs should be avoided since they increase risk of GI bleeds, can cause renal impairment and can result in fluid retention (which will worsen a patient's ascites).

Sedative and constipating drugs should be used cautiously since they may precipitate hepatic encephalopathy.

Drugs that are metabolised by the liver may accumulate in liver disease and thus may require dose reductions.

11. **Which drug would be the best option for the management of the following problems in a patient with liver disease:**
- **pain associated with a sprained ankle?**
  Paracetamol may be used, but halve the dose. If ineffective, a low dose of opioid may be given (providing the patient is not encephalopathic), e.g. codeine 30 mg two or three times daily. Laxatives should be prescribed to avoid constipation.
- **depression?**
  Paroxetine is recommended due to its shorter elimination half-life.
- **epilepsy?**
  Phenytoin is the drug of choice, but a lower dose will be required due to reduced hepatic metabolism and serum albumin (phenytoin binds to albumin).

NP Neurology and psychiatry

Chapter contents

The assistance of Mr David Kitchen MSc MRPharmS, Principal Pharmacist, MerseyCare NHS Trust, in the preparation of this section is gratefully acknowledged.

Introduction

Although neurological and psychiatric morbidity covers a wide range of problems, many of which require specialist care, three of the most commonly encountered problems are discussed here.

Problem 1: the patient has depression

Depression is often both undertreated and over-treated. As with other psychiatric disorders, there is a complex interaction between mind and body which means that drug therapy can only be a part of the treatment, and sometimes is not indicated at all. However, when it is used there is good evidence that it is effective in resolving depression in most patients.

Problem 2: the patient has Parkinson's disease

This degenerative disease, characterised by problems initiating voluntary movement, tremor, rigidity and changes in gait, is due to a deficiency in dopaminergic neurons in the basal ganglia of the brain. Several lines of pharmacological therapy have been developed, but the exact place of each in therapy is still unclear. NICE guidance is awaited in 2006 but the major controversy in therapy relates to the decision as to whether levodopa therapy should be initiated early or late. This is affected by the age and condition of the patient.

Problem 3: the patient has epilepsy

Epilepsy, like Parkinson's disease, requires specialist diagnosis and management. The application of drug therapy is illustrated with reference to the management of tonic–clonic seizure control, though it contains principles common to the other forms. These include reducing the number of attacks, avoidance of adverse events from drug therapy and managing drug interactions.

The pharmacist's role

This is a diverse group of conditions, drawn from a much wider possible selection to illustrate the range of neurological and psychiatric morbidity. All these conditions may leave patients feeling embarrassment and social stigma in a way that other ill-health might not. They are treated with drug therapy that can be effective in many patients and yet often it is poorly tolerated and creates new problems, including adverse events and interaction potential. Pharmacists should remember that in psychiatric illness there may be difficulties in comprehension and complying with therapy. It is especially important to remember that your first responsibility is to the patient, and for listeners to take on board what the patient is saying to ensure concordance between patient, doctor and pharmacist.

Neurology and psychiatry 1 problem: the patient has depression

 Objectives of this section

The reader should be able to detail:
- the objectives of care in depression
- how GPs recognise depression and classify it by severity
- the importance of non-drug measures, especially in mild depression and dysthymia (persistently lowered mood)
- the importance of promoting compliance in achieving resolution
- the main treatment options available:
  — tricyclic antidepressants
  — selective serotonin reuptake inhibitors (SSRIs)
  — newer antidepressants, and their place in therapy
- monitoring required to ensure safety and efficacy of drug therapy.

 Further reading: basics

- *British National Formulary*, current edn. London: Royal Pharmaceutical Society and British Medical Association. Section 4.3: Antidepressant drugs. (ONLINE)
- Randall MD, Neil KE. *Disease Management*. London: Pharmaceutical Press; 2004. Chapter 23: Affective disorders.

 Further reading: moving on

- Walker R, Edwards C, eds. *Clinical Pharmacy and Therapeutics*, 3rd edn. London: Churchill

Livingstone; 2003. Chapter 27: Affective disorders.
- Dodds LJ, ed. *Drugs in Use*, 3rd edn. London: Pharmaceutical Press; 2003. Chapter 18: Depression.

 Guidelines

- National Institute for Clinical Excellence. *Clinical Guideline 23: Management of Depression in Primary and Secondary Care.* London: NICE; 2004. (ONLINE)

 Self-assessment questions: Neurology and psychiatry 1
(Answers on p. 109)

1. Why should mild depression be treated first with non-drug therapy?
2. What markers indicate that a patient may be suffering from depression?
3. Which drugs should be the first-choice therapy in depression once therapy is initiated?
4. Do SSRIs offer any advantages over tricyclic antidepressants (TCAs) in the management of depression?
5. What if the patient does not respond?
6. What place does St John's wort *(Hypericum perforatum)* have in the management of depression?
7. Why do the NICE guidelines recommend the avoidance of dosulepin (dothiepin) and venlafaxine as initial choices of drug therapy?
8. What counselling is required when a patient commences antidepressant therapy?
9. What less common adverse events are shared by all types of antidepressants?
10. When can treatment be stopped?
11. When should specialist referral be obtained?

Chart 2.18 Neurology and psychiatry 1 problem: the patient has depression

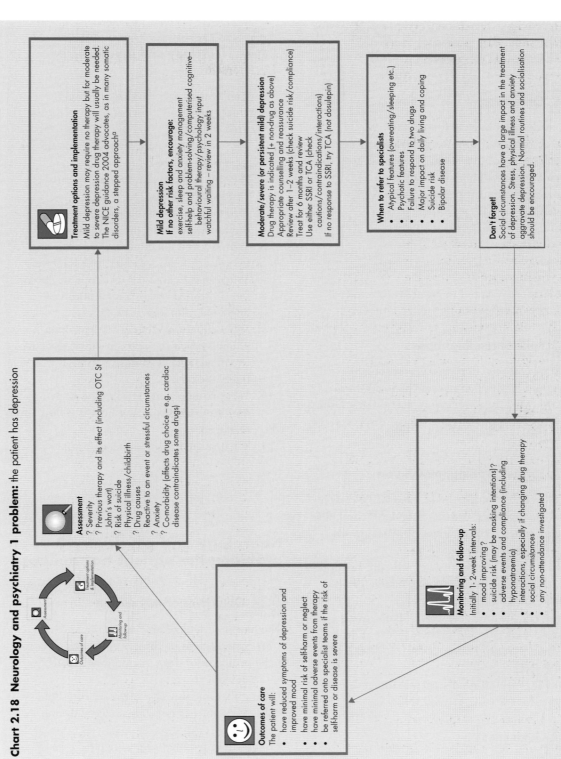

Treatment options and implementation

Mild depression may require no therapy but for moderate to severe depression drug therapy will usually be needed. The NICE guidance 2004 advocates, as in many somatic disorders, a stepped approach[a]

Mild depression
If no other risk factors, encourage:
exercise, sleep and anxiety management
self-help and problem-solving/computerised cognitive–behavioural therapy/psychology input
watchful waiting – review in 2 weeks

Moderate/severe (or persistent mild) depression
Drug therapy is indicated (+ non-drug as above)
Appropriate counselling and reassurance
Review after 1–2 weeks (check suicide risk/compliance)
Treat for 6 months and review
Use either SSRI or TCA (check cautions/contraindications/interactions)
If no response to SSRI, try TCA (not dosulepin)

When to refer to specialists
• Atypical features (overeating/sleeping etc.)
• Psychotic features
• Failure to respond to two drugs
• Major impact on daily living and coping
• Suicide risk
• Bipolar disease

Don't forget!
Social circumstances have a large impact in the treatment of depression. Stress, physical illness and anxiety aggravate depression. Normal routines and socialisation should be encouraged.

Assessment
? Severity
? Previous therapy and its effect (including OTC St John's wort)
? Risk of suicide
? Physical illness/childbirth
? Drug causes
? Reactive to an event or stressful circumstances
? Anxiety
? Co-morbidity (affects drug choice – e.g. cardiac disease contraindicates some drugs)

Outcomes of care
The patient will:
• have reduced symptoms of depression and improved mood
• have minimal risk of self-harm or neglect
• have minimal adverse events from therapy
• be referred onto specialist teams if the risk of self-harm or disease is severe

Monitoring and follow-up
Initially 1- 2-week intervals:
• mood improving?
• suicide risk (may be masking intentions)?
• adverse events and compliance (including hyponatraemia)
• interactions, especially if changing drug therapy
• social circumstances
• any non-attendance investigated

Assessment

Treatment options & implementation

Monitoring and follow-up

Outcomes of care

[a]National Institute for Clinical Excellence. Clinical Excellence. Clinical Guideline 23: Management of Depression in Primary and Secondary Care. London: NICE; 2004. (ONLINE)

Neurology and psychiatry 2 problem: the patient has Parkinson's disease

 Objectives of this section

The reader should be able to detail:
- the objectives of care in Parkinson's disease
- the importance of treating associated problems such as depression and constipation
- the main treatment options available:
  — levodopa (with a peripheral dopa-decarboxylase inhibitor)
  — dopamine agonists
  — selegiline
  — entacapone
- monitoring required to ensure safety and efficacy of drug therapy.

 Further reading: basics

- *British National Formulary*, current edn. London: Royal Pharmaceutical Society and British Medical Association. Section 4.9: Drugs used in parkinsonism and related disorders. (ONLINE)

 Further reading: moving on

- Walker R, Edwards C, eds. *Clinical Pharmacy and Therapeutics*, 3rd edn. London: Churchill Livingstone; 2003. Chapter 30: Parkinson's disease.
- Dodds LJ, ed. *Drugs in Use*, 3rd edn. London: Pharmaceutical Press; 2003. Chapter 15: Parkinson's disease.
- Chan KL, Jagait P, Tugwell C. Parkinson's disease – current and future aspects of drug treatment. *Hosp Pharm* 2004; 11: 18–22. (ONLINE)
- Burn D. Parkinson's disease: treatment. *Pharm J* 2000; 264: 476–479. (ONLINE)

 Guidelines

- NICE guidance awaited.

 Self-assessment questions: Neurology and psychiatry 2
(Answers on p. 112)

1. Can drugs cause Parkinson's disease?
2. Does Parkinson's disease always require drug therapy?
3. Why is therapy with levodopa not always used immediately?
4. What treatments are suitable in early Parkinson's disease?
5. What approach should be taken if the disease has become more symptomatic?
6. Why is levodopa administered with a peripheral dopa-decarboxylase inhibitor?
7. When should doses of levodopa be taken?
8. Do controlled release preparations of levodopa offer any advantages?
9. What should be done when levodopa patients reach the point at which they are experiencing end-of-dose response fluctuations?
10. What co-morbidity is common in Parkinson's disease, and how is it best managed?
11. What is the role of apomorphine?

Neurology and psychiatry 3 problem: the patient has epilepsy

 Objectives of this section

The reader should be able to detail:
- the management of chronic epilepsy
- the problems of drug interactions involving antiepileptic drugs
- drugs that may lower the seizure threshold
- the problems of managing epilepsy during pregnancy
- monitoring required to ensure efficacy and safety of therapy.

Chart 2.19 Neurology and psychiatry 2 problem: the patient has Parkinson's disease

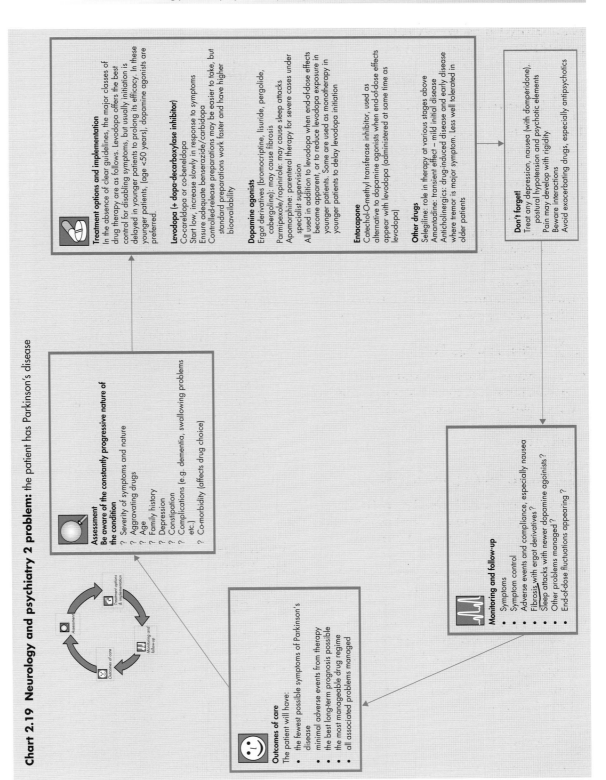

Assessment

Be aware of the constantly progressive nature of the condition

? Severity of symptoms and nature
? Aggravating drugs
? Age
? Family history
? Depression
? Constipation
? Complications (e.g. dementia, swallowing problems etc.)
? Co-morbidity (affects drug choice)

Treatment options and implementation

In the absence of clear guidelines, the major classes of drug therapy are as follows. Levodopa offers the best control for disabling symptoms, but usually initiation is delayed in younger patients to prolong its efficacy. In these younger patients, (age <50 years), dopamine agonists are preferred.

Levodopa (+ dopa-decarboxylase inhibitor)

Co-careldopa or co-beneldopa
Start low, increase slowly in response to symptoms
Ensure adequate benserazide/carbidopa
Controlled-release preparations may be easier to take, but standard preparations work faster and have higher bioavailability

Dopamine agonists

Ergot derivatives (bromocriptine, lisuride, pergolide, cabergoline): may cause fibrosis
Parmipexole/ropinirole: may cause sleep attacks
Apomorphine: parenteral therapy for severe cases under specialist supervision
All used in addition to levodopa when end-of-dose effects become apparent, or to reduce levodopa exposure in younger patients. Some are used as monotherapy in younger patients to delay levodopa initiation

Entacapone

Catechol-O-methyl transferase inhibitor, used as alternative to dopamine agonists when end-of-dose effects appear with levodopa (administered at same time as levodopa)

Other drugs

Selegiline: role in therapy at various stages above
Amantadine: transient effect – mild initial disease
Anticholinergics: drug-induced disease and early disease where tremor is major symptom. Less well tolerated in older patients

Don't forget!

Treat any depression, nausea (with domperidone), postural hypotension and psychotic elements
Pain may develop with rigidity
Beware interactions
Avoid exacerbating drugs, especially antipsychotics

Monitoring and follow-up

• Symptoms
• Symptom control
• Adverse events and compliance, especially nausea
• Fibrosis with ergot derivatives ?
• Sleep attacks with newer dopamine agonists ?
• Other problems managed ?
• End-of-dose fluctuations appearing ?

Outcomes of care

The patient will have:

• the fewest possible symptoms of Parkinson's disease
• minimal adverse events from therapy
• the best long-term prognosis possible
• the most manageable drug regime
• all associated problems managed

Chart 2.20 Neurology and psychiatry 3 problem: the patient has epilepsy

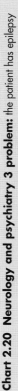

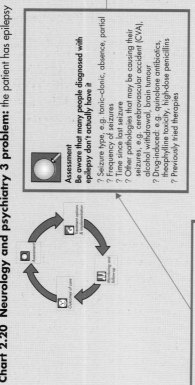

Treatment options and implementation

Initiation of treatment follows confirmation of the diagnosis of epilepsy and is generally recommended after a second epileptic seizure. The choice of agent depends upon the type of seizures experienced. Since tonic–clonic seizures are the most common type encountered, the treatment of these is discussed here.

General principles of the chronic management of tonic–clonic seizures (NICE guidance)[a]

- Monotherapy is preferred where possible
- If the first agent fails, try monotherapy with another drug
- Use combination therapy after attempts with monotherapy have failed to achieve adequate long-term control
- When switching to another agent, titrate the new drug to the maximum tolerated dose, then slowly withdraw the previous drug

Choice of agent

- First-line agents: carbamazepine, sodium valproate, lamotrigine, topiramate
- Second-line agents: clobazam, levetiracetam, oxcarbazepine
- Benzodiazepines (clonazepam and clobazam) are used for short-term cover of, for example, weddings and exams
- Other agents to consider: phenobarbital, phenytoin, primidone
- Avoid tiagabine and vigabatrin – may worsen tonic–clonic seizures

Assessment

Be aware that many people diagnosed with epilepsy don't actually have it

- ? Seizure type, e.g. tonic–clonic, absence, partial
- ? Frequency of seizures
- ? Time since last seizure
- ? Other pathologies that may be causing their seizures, e.g. cerebrovascular accident (CVA), alcohol withdrawal, brain tumour
- ? Drug-induced: e.g. quinolone antibiotics, theophylline toxicity, high-dose penicillins
- ? Previously tried therapies

Don't forget!

- Differences in bioavailability exist between different brands and preparations, so patients should be maintained on the same brand and formulation, e.g. Tegretol Retard
- Many of the anticonvulsants are hepatically metabolised and have the potential for drug interactions. Levels of both the anticonvulsants themselves and other prescribed therapies may be affected and require close monitoring
- Compliance with anticonvulsant therapy is often poor due to adverse effects but often simply failure to remember to take a 'preventive' medication
- No need to take anticonvulsants more than twice a day
- Epileptic patients are required to inform the DVLA when they have a seizure and must be seizure-free for at least a year before they may re-apply for their driving licence
- There are a number of drugs that may lower the seizure threshold, e.g. quinolone antibiotics and antidepressants. Whilst not all of these are contraindicated in a patient with epilepsy, careful consideration of the risks versus the benefits of such additional therapy is required
- Many of the anticonvulsants are teratogenic. However, poorly controlled epilepsy also represents a risk to the fetus. Pregnant patients require specialist care
- Oral contraceptives may be affected by anticonvulsants

Monitoring and follow-up

- Frequency of seizures
- LFTs (e.g. for carbamazepine, sodium valproate)
- FBC: dyscrasias with carbamazepine and valproate
- Side-effects, e.g. sedation
- Plasma concentrations for phenytoin, phenobarbital, carbamazepine
- Patient compliance
- Patient's perception of therapy

Outcomes of care

The patient will have:
- reduced incidence of seizures
- minimal side-effects from their medication
- potential drug interactions managed appropriately
- an improved quality of life

[a]National Institute for Clinical Excellence. *Clinical Guideline 20: The Epilepsies: The diagnosis and management of the epilepsies in adults and children in primary and secondary care.* London: NICE; 2004. (ONLINE)

Further reading: basics

- *British National Formulary*, current edn. London: Royal Pharmaceutical Society and British Medical Association. Section 4.8: Antiepileptics. (ONLINE)
- Randall MD, Neil KE. *Disease Management*. London: Pharmaceutical Press; 2004. Chapter 22: Epilepsy.

 Further reading: moving on

- Walker R, Edwards C, eds. *Clinical Pharmacy and Therapeutics*, 3rd edn. London: Churchill Livingstone; 2003. Chapter 29: Epilepsy.
- Dodds LJ, ed. *Drugs in Use*, 3rd edn. London: Pharmaceutical Press; 2003. Chapter 14: Epilepsy.

 Guidelines

- National Institute for Clinical Excellence. *Clinical Guideline 20: The Epilepsies: The diagnosis and management of the epilepsies in adults and children in primary and secondary care.* London: NICE; 2004. (ONLINE)

 Self-assessment questions: Neurology and psychiatry 3
(Answers on p. 114)

1. A young female patient has had repeated tonic–clonic seizures and is commenced on phenytoin 300 mg od. What would be your response?
2. A patient is to be started on carbamazepine. How should this drug be introduced and the dose titrated?
3. A patient is receiving carbamazepine 200 mg bd for tonic–clonic seizures, but develops a severe erythematous rash. What action should be taken?
4. Which anticonvulsants are generally considered to be the safest to use during pregnancy?
5. During a ward round a female patient is commenced on ciprofloxacin 500 mg bd for a urinary tract infection (UTI). Her other medication consists of carbamazepine 400 mg bd. What would your response be?
6. A patient enters your community pharmacy and requests St John's wort. After further questioning you discover that they also take carbamazepine 600 mg bd. How would you deal with this request?

 Answers to self-assessment questions: Neurology and psychiatry 1: depression (p. 104)

1. **Why should mild depression be treated first with non-drug therapy?**
   This is essentially a question of risk–benefit. Mild depression often resolves spontaneously and is also amenable to various non-drug therapies. In the first instance this may consist of removal from stressful situations, adopting a structured exercise regime, and trying to sleep longer and better. GPs can back this up with computerised cognitive–behavioural therapy, directed self-help material or referral to psychological services, though there is a

(Continued)

correlation between the quality of the psychological interaction and its effect. This may resolve a low mood quickly with no need to initiate drug therapy. In patients at low risk of deterioration, self-harm or neglect of themselves or others, a review in a couple of weeks may be scheduled. If this is so, the patient needs a source of help if they suddenly feel worse, and to be sought out if they do not return.

2. **What markers indicate that a patient may be suffering from depression?**
Many guidelines have lists of markers of depression or scoring systems contained within them, but the same result may be obtained in most patients by asking two questions such as:
   - asking about mood over the last month
   - asking about affect – interest and enjoyment in doing things over the last month.

In addition, the patient should always be asked about the likelihood of them harming themselves, in a manner that encourages an honest response

3. **Which drugs should be the first-choice therapy in depression once therapy is initiated?**
Efficacy, tolerability and cost mean that the two main standard therapies are using TCAs or SSRIs. The NICE guidance in 2004 suggests that SSRIs should be preferred because of a reduced risk of discontinuation due to adverse events, but the difference is probably not large. There are many SSRIs available now, and probably all have similar efficacy, but fluoxetine defines the class, is available generically and has a lower rate of withdrawal symptoms. Citalopram is another recommended first choice with fewer drug interactions. Sertraline is better evidenced in cardiac disease. The guidelines suggest that primary care and non-specialist

teams should avoid using venlafaxine and dosulepin (dothiepin), and also reserve the addition of lithium or use of monoamine oxidase inhibitors (MAOIs) to specialists, who might include some GPs.

4. **Do SSRIs offer any advantages over TCAs in the management of depression?**
In addition to a reduced risk of withdrawal, SSRIs are much safer than TCAs in overdose. With the exception of lofepramine, the antimuscarinic side-effects of TCAs can be extremely cardiotoxic in overdose. Many of the SSRIs are initiated at their normal maximum dose, whereas TCAs need titration upwards over time, which may lead to delays in getting the condition under control. Finally SSRIs are less sedating than many of the TCAs, which can be an advantage, though insomnia may respond better to a sedating drug. The risk of restlessness, agitation, nausea and suicidal ideation may be greater with SSRIs.

5. **What if the patient does not respond?**
Compliance should be checked, and the dosage reviewed if the patient does not begin to improve in 3–4 weeks. It may be that there are higher doses that can be used within the product licence. Older people may take longer to respond. If a partial response is obtained, the drug can be tried for 6 weeks. However, at that point, if not sooner, an alternative therapy can be tried, although interactions should be observed for – many of these drugs have long half-lives. SSRIs can be substituted with an alternative SSRI, though serotonin syndrome should be monitored for (chills, confusion, spasms). A TCA (with dose titration) is a reasonable alternative if suitable, and NICE recommends consideration of moclobemide (a reversible inhibitor of MAOI type A), after a washout period, or reboxetine

$\rightarrow$

(noradrenaline reuptake inhibitor with fewer long-term safety data).

6. **What place does St John's wort (*Hypericum perforatum*) have in the management of depression?**

No licensed preparations of this herbal remedy exist and so there is variability in the products available, but it is effective in mild depression. It is an inducer of metabolising enzymes in the liver, leading to a series of interactions with metabolised drugs as described in the *BNF*, including antidepressants, and so concomitant use is best avoided. For patients with mild depression who wish to purchase this product as an alternative to starting conventional therapies, it may offer benefits. It must not, however, be used as a substitute for prescription remedies in the more severely depressed.

7. **Why do the NICE guidelines recommend the avoidance of dosulepin (dothiepin) and venlafaxine as initial choices of drug therapy?**

Dothiepin was formerly very popular with GPs, as it was well tolerated, but it seems more cardiotoxic and dangerous in overdose than the other TCAs. Venlafaxine, a serotonin and noradrenaline reuptake inhibitor, is restricted by NICE to patients who have tried two other therapies, and have no pre-existing cardiac disease. It is more expensive, more toxic in overdose and more liable to cause withdrawal due to adverse events than the SSRIs. An ECG and blood pressure measurement is needed before commencing therapy. However, any doctor can prescribe it and it has become popular, due to some evidence that it is effective in refractory cases.

8. **What counselling is required when a patient commences antidepressant therapy?**

The patient needs to be treated sympathetically and with empathy, as their self-esteem may be low and there is a stigma associated with psychiatric morbidity. They need to understand that the treatment may take a month or more to relieve symptoms, whereas any adverse events may present much more quickly, so concordance is important to promote compliance. Suicide ideation is greatest early in therapy, and a review date and appointment must be given, and non-attendance followed up. Stressing that antidepressants are non-addictive may help compliance, but patients should be warned that some drugs have withdrawal syndromes if stopped too quickly, and the depression may recur if 6 months or more therapy has not been taken.

Patient information leaflets will contain a lot of information about contraindications, cautions, interactions and adverse events, and if the patient feels that any of these have been overlooked before the drug was prescribed this will impair compliance. Stressing that there is hope and that the drugs are usually effective will be helpful.

9. **What less common adverse events are shared by all types of antidepressants?**

Hyponatraemia, especially with elderly people, due to inappropriate secretion of antidiuretic hormone, is common to most antidepressants, and probably more so with SSRIs. Similarly, antidepressants from both main groups can lower the seizure threshold, which is particulary risky in people with epilepsy.

10. **When can treatment be stopped?**

Most sources suggest that, if remission is achieved, therapy should be continued for at least 6 months. At that point review may suggest that therapy can be stopped. Some drugs are associated with withdrawal symptoms, so reduction of dose (if possible) or frequency is advised over several weeks as an intermediate measure. If a patient has

(Continued)

had recurrent or disabling depression, treatment may be necessary for two or more years.

11. **When should specialist referral be obtained?**
Patients who have not responded to two drugs, who are severely disabled or at risk of suicide, or who have recurrent or persistent depression or other complicating factors need referral or extra support. In most parts of the country this will be delivered by specialists with access to inpatient care, community support, psychological programmes and the knowledge to prescribe a wider range of therapies.

 Answers to self-assessment questions:
Neurology and psychiatry 2: Parkinson's disease (p. 106)

1. **Can drugs cause Parkinson's disease?**
The extrapyramidal side-effects of antipsychotic therapy are well recognised, including those of closely related drugs such as prochlorperazine and cinnarizine. Lithium, MAOIs, amiodarone and some CCBs as well as other therapies have also been implicated. The drug should be withdrawn and usually the condition will resolve over weeks to months. However, it may recur and it is thought that this is because the offending drug had exposed a pre-clinical parkinsonism.

2. **Does Parkinson's disease always require drug therapy?**
No. Early disease, with non-disabling symptoms, may simply require reassurance and lifestyle changes. There is no evidence that early treatment will improve the overall prognosis, and since the drugs carry a high rate of adverse events then it may be better to delay initiating therapy.

3. **Why is therapy with levodopa not always used immediately?**
Levodopa, in combination with peripheral dopa-decarboxylase inhibitors, is certainly the most effective therapy to control the disabling symptoms of Parkinson's disease. However, about 10% of the patients prescribed it lose full responsiveness to it each year. Specifically, as the dose wears off the patient fluctuates between jerky movements (dyskinesias) and rigidity, sometimes called 'on-offing' or 'yo-yoing.' At 10 years into therapy, virtually all patients have these problems. As this evidence has emerged, there has been a tendency to 'spare' levodopa by initiating it later, especially in younger patients. Alternatively, lower doses may be possible by using the levodopa in combination with another drug. Many younger patients will thus be more appropriately commenced on dopamine agonists as initial therapy.

4. **What treatments are suitable in early Parkinson's disease?**
The initial symptoms of Parkinson's disease often include tremor, and these are manageable with the anticholinergic drugs such as trihexyphenidyl (benzhexol), and others. Amantadine, formerly used to treat influenza, may have a place because it is well tolerated, but its effect is only transient. Finally, the MAOI type B, selegiline, is still preferred by many specialists.

5. **What approach should be taken if the disease has become more symptomatic?**
If the patient is suffering from disabling symptoms, especially if they are elderly (and therefore not likely to have to take the therapy for as long as a younger sufferer), it may be perfectly appropriate to start

→

levodopa therapy. However, the trend seems to have moved in recent years to delay initiation in younger patients, for the reasons discussed above. In these patients a centrally acting dopamine agonist is the preferred therapy, with more drugs than previously was the case becoming licensed for monotherapy and early initiation. Levodopa can then be added in later once the dopamine agonist is unable to control the disease symptoms.

6. **Why is the levodopa administered with a peripheral dopa-decarboxylase inhibitor?**
The only licensed levodopa preparations in the UK contain either benserazide (co-beneldopa) or carbidopa (co-careldopa). All co-beneldopa preparations contain the same ratio of benserazide to levodopa but the co-careldopa preparations come in different ratios. The presence of the dopa-decarboxylase inhibitor prevents the levodopa being converted into dopamine in the peripheral circulation. This would not only reduce the availability of levodopa in the central nervous system (CNS), but also cause more adverse events such as nausea. The levodopa gets into the CNS and is eventually used as a precursor of dopamine, a very water-soluble, short-lived (*in vivo*) compound that cannot be administered to treat Parkinson's disease in any useful manner. The peripheral dopa-decarboxylase inhibitor does not cross the blood–brain barrier. Unfortunately the daily dose of benserazide or carbidopa required to suppress dopa-decarboxylase is 70–100 mg, and lower doses of the combination products (used especially when initiating therapy) may not provide enough enzyme inhibitor.

7. **When should doses of levodopa be taken?**
Most patients benefit from taking their levodopa with food. The slower absorption reduces adverse events by reducing the post-dose peak in blood level. However, patients on large doses of levodopa as the disease progresses may not be able to do this. The higher blood levels are needed to control the disease.

8. **Do controlled release preparations of levodopa offer any advantages?**
It was thought that they might correct the end-of-dose symptoms, but in practice it seems that their major benefit is to simplify regimes. The patient often has a supply of short-acting tablets to take when the fluctuations begin, or when they awake rigid – these will work a lot more quickly than controlled-release preparations. Given the range of preparations available with sometimes ambiguous names, great care should be taken to ensure that the patient receives the correct formulation. If controlled-release preparations are used, a dose increase will be required to correct for their lower bioavailability.

9. **What should be done when levodopa patients reach the point at which they are experiencing end-of-dose response fluctuations?**
There are two main options. The first, and until recently the only real choice, was to select a direct dopamine agonist. These fall into two groups: those based on ergot (bromocriptine, cabergoline, lisuride and pergolide), and pramipexole and ropinerole. The ergot derivatives can cause fibrotic reactions, and monitoring for cough, chest or abdominal pain, and heart failure is needed. The other two drugs are safer in this regard but can cause attacks of somnolence, of sudden falling asleep with little warning, and patients who drive need to be warned of this, if they have not already had to surrender their licences to the Driver and Vehicle Licensing Agency (DVLA).

(Continued)

An alternative strategy is to use the catechol-O-methyl transferase inhibitor entacapone. This slows the breakdown of both dopamine in the CNS and levodopa in the peripheral circulation. Entacapone is reasonably well tolerated and available as both tablets and a combined preparation with levodopa and carbidopa. It seems likely that doctors will increasingly try entacapone in place of the dopamine agonist as the add-on to levodopa when this is no longer sufficient – but a reduction in levodopa dose is needed.

10. **What co-morbidity is common in Parkinson's disease, and how is it best managed?**
Nausea is usually a result of drugs that act to increase dopamine levels, and is best treated with domperidone, a dopamine antagonist that does not cross the blood–brain barrier (as metoclopramide does) and thus will not aggravate Parkinson's disease symptoms. Constipation is an adverse event of drugs as well as a manifestation of the disease and will respond to diet and fluids and, if required, laxatives. Psychotic problems may be aggravated by the adverse effects of dopaminergic therapy. Finally depression is commonly seen, and can be safely managed with SSRIs. Although TCAs may help other problems such as drooling, care should be taken to avoid exacerbating hypotension. If a patient is taking selegiline, there will be interactions with the antidepressant – guidance is in the *BNF*.

11. **What is the role of apomorphine?**
Apomorphine is an extremely potent dopamine agonist although, since it can be given only parenterally and is very irritant, administration is not easy, nor is it cheap. However, in patients who are losing response to other drugs it can be a near-miracle therapy and a variety of infusion techniques are available to administer it. Extreme nausea means that therapy must be preceded by 3 days' administration of high-dose domperidone. Expert advice is always necessary to optimise therapy.

 Answers to self-assessment questions:
Neurology and psychiatry 3: epilepsy (p. 109)

1. **A young female patient has had repeated tonic–clonic seizures and is commenced on phenytoin 300 mg od. What would be your response?**
Phenytoin is no longer the first-choice treatment for the long-term management of epilepsy. The drug is associated with many unpleasant side-effects, including hirsutism and gingival hyperplasia. In addition, phenytoin follows zero-order pharmacokinetics, which makes dosing more difficult. The first-line treatment would be lamotrigine, sodium valproate or carbamazepine.

2. **A patient is to be started on carbamazepine. How should this drug be introduced and the dose titrated?**
The dose of carbamazepine needs gradual titration to minimise dose-related side-effects, e.g. dizziness, drowsiness and visual disturbances. It should also be noted that carbamazepine induces its own metabolism. Carbamazepine is initiated at a dose 100–200 mg once or twice daily, increasing in increments of 100–200 mg every 2 weeks to a usual dose of 800–1200 mg daily in divided doses.

→

3. **A patient is receiving carbamazepine 200 mg bd for tonic–clonic seizures, but develops a severe erythematous rash. What action should be taken?**

This is a well-reported ADR associated with carbamazepine use. However, before any action is taken it is essential that other possible causes of the rash be excluded. If the rash is due to the carbamazepine, an alternative anticonvulsant is required. Suitable alternatives include sodium valproate, lamotrigine, topiramate and levetiracetam. If it was not for the rash, the carbamazepine dose would be reduced gradually over several weeks (after the new agent has been titrated to a therapeutic dose), but in this case the specialist may wish to reduce the dose more rapidly.

4. **Which anticonvulsants are generally considered to be the safest to use during pregnancy?**

No single anticonvulsant is deemed 100% safe to use during pregnancy. Carbamazepine, oxcarbazepine, phenytoin and sodium valproate are associated with a higher risk of neural tube defects than the newer agents. The benefits versus the risks of treatment need to be considered carefully in all these patients. Folic acid supplementation (before and during pregnancy) may reduce the risk of neural tube defects if the patient needs to remain on their anticonvulsant therapy.

5. **During a ward round a female patient is commenced on ciprofloxacin 500 mg bd for a UTI. Her other medication consists of carbamazepine 400 mg bd. What would your response be?**

Since carbamazepine may be used for both epilepsy and neuropathic pain, it is important to determine the indication for which the patient is taking the carbamazepine. Ciprofloxacin is a quinolone antibiotic, which can lower the seizure threshold and should be avoided where possible in a patient with epilepsy. Suitable alternatives for a patient with epilepsy would be trimethoprim, cephalexin or co-amoxiclav – depending on cultures and sensitivities and patient allergies.

6. **A patient enters your community pharmacy and requests St John's wort. After further questioning you discover that they also take carbamazepine 600 mg bd. How would you deal with this request?**

St John's wort induces the metabolism of carbamazepine, can significantly reduce plasma concentrations and should thus be avoided in patients receiving carbamazepine therapy. The patient should be referred to their GP if they feel depressed – the use of antidepressant therapy in epileptic patients also requires caution since antidepressants may lower the seizure threshold.

SG Surgical and general problems

Chapter contents

The assistance of Mr Mohamed Rahman MSc MRPharmS, Principal Pharmacist, Surgical Services at the Royal Liverpool and Broadgreen University Hospitals NHS Trust, in the preparation of this section is gratefully acknowledged.

 Problem 1: the patient is to have surgery

Patients requiring surgery frequently require a pharmacist's input. Their usual medication may have to be withheld or changed prior to surgery. The patient may also be nil by mouth for a prolonged period of time, which will impact on the administration of medication. Certain co-morbidities, e.g. diabetes, CVD, will require special consideration. There are also a number of potential complications associated with surgery which may be prevented (e.g. infection, thrombembolism, nausea and pain).

 Problem 2: the patient requires intravenous fluids or nutrition

Fluid replacement therapy may be required by a variety of patients. Patients who undergo surgery are at risk of dehydration due to them being unable to take oral fluids, losses during surgery and losses from fistulae/drains. Dehydration is also a complication of many different diseases and may result in patients being admitted to hospital.

 Problem 3: the patient requires palliative care

Palliative care aims to provide relief from suffering and improve the quality of a patient's life in the final stages of an incurable disease. A holistic approach is taken which combines physical, psychological, social and spiritual care. Attention must also be given to the patient's relatives, friends and carers during this time. During the terminal phases of a patient's illness, they may be unable to take anything orally, which impacts on drug administration.

 Problem 4: the patient has had a thromboembolic event

A thromboembolism can present as either a deep vein thrombosis which may move to the lung and result in a pulmonary embolism, or the direct formation of a pulmonary embolus which, if untreated, carries significant mortality. The initial treatment involves heparin, followed by warfarin therapy once the diagnosis is confirmed (which requires close monitoring). The patient will also require any risk factors for thromboembolism to be identified, some of which can be modified to prevent recurrence of this event.

The pharmacist's role

Many patients requiring surgery have other co-morbidities which can affect their management during the perioperative period. The pharmacist has a crucial role to play in providing advice regarding the management of the patient during this period. Patients receiving palliative care may be experiencing numerous symptoms requiring drug therapy, on which the pharmacist can advise. When syringe drivers are used, the pharmacist can advise on stability of mixtures of drugs. Since warfarin therapy can be dangerous if not managed properly, pharmacists have an important role to play in patient counselling and may even be involved with the running of anticoagulant clinics.

Surgical and general 1 problem: the patient is to have surgery

 Objectives of this section

The reader should be able to detail:
- the objectives of care in patients who are to have surgery
- the management of the patient in the peri-operative period
- the common postoperative complications and how they may be prevented and managed:
  — thromboembolism
  — infection
  — pain

— nausea and vomiting
— constipation
— dehydration
- monitoring required to ensure efficacy and safety of drug therapy.

 Further reading: basics

- *British National Formulary*, current edn. London: Royal Pharmaceutical Society and British Medical Association. Sections 15: Anaesthesia and 4.7: Analgesics. (ONLINE)
- Walker R, Edwards C, eds. *Clinical Pharmacy and Therapeutics*, 3rd edn. London: Churchill Livingstone; 2003. Chapters 31: Pain; and 32: Nausea and vomiting.
- Dodds LJ, ed. *Drugs in Use*, 3rd edn. London: Pharmaceutical Press; 2003. Chapter 29: Colorectal surgery.

 Further reading: moving on

- Rahman M, Beattie J. Medication in the peri-operative period. *Pharm J* 2004; 272: 287–289. (ONLINE)
- Rahman M, Beattie J. Peri-operative care and diabetes. *Pharm J* 2004; 272: 323–325. (ONLINE)
- Rahman M, Beattie J. Peri-operative medication in patients with cardiovascular disease. *Pharm J* 2004; 272: 352–354. (ONLINE)
- Rahman M, Anson J. Peri-operative antibiotic prophylaxis. *Pharm J* 2004; 272: 743–745. (ONLINE)
- Rahman M, Beattie J. Drugs used to prevent surgical VTE. *Pharm J* 2004; 273: 717–719. (ONLINE)
- Rahman M, Beattie J. Post-operative nausea and vomiting. *Pharm J* 2004; 273: 786–788. (ONLINE)
- Rahman M, Beattie J. Managing post-operative pain. *Pharm J* 2005; 275: 145–148. (ONLINE)

Chart 2.21 Surgical and general 1 problem: the patient is to have surgery

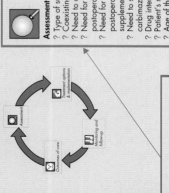

Assessment

- ? Type of surgery the patient is to have
- ? Coexisting medical problems (co-morbidities)
- ? Need to continue current drug treatments
- ? Need for new medication (for short-term treatment) postoperatively, e.g. analgesics, anti-emetics
- ? Need for new medication (for long-term treatment) postoperatively, e.g. calcium and vitamin D supplements after a parathyroidectomy
- ? Need to stop medication postoperatively, e.g. carbimazole following a thyroidectomy
- ? Patient's renal function
- ? Age of the patient
- ? Duration of period of immobility
- ? Duration that patient is to be nil by mouth (NBM)
- ? Prophylactic antibiotics prescribed/needed

Treatment options and implementation

It is vital that all of the patient's usual medication is continued where appropriate – the medicines being taken and the type of surgery the patient will have will influence this.
The approaches used to reduce postoperative complications will again depend on the type of surgery.

Problems associated with surgery

- Ensure all of the patient's usual medication is prescribed where appropriate (see BNF)
- Avoid postoperative thromboembolism
- Avoid surgical site infection
- Treat postoperative pain effectively while minimising side-effects
- Prevent/treat postoperative nausea and vomiting effectively, as appropriate
- Treat constipation
- Avoid postoperative dehydration or fluid overload
- Wound management
- Impact of surgery on a patient's nutritional status (e.g. after small bowel resections or pancreatic surgery)

Don't forget!

There are some groups of patients who require special attention when they have surgery:

- people with diabetes – will require conversion of SC insulin to IV insulin. Patients with type 2 diabetes receiving oral hypoglycaemics may also require IV insulin therapy
- patients with cardiovascular disease
- patients taking long-term steroids will require additional doses of hydrocortisone on the day of surgery since they will be unable to mount an adequate stress response to the surgery
- patients taking antidepressants, e.g. MAOIs
- patients prescribed either the oral contraceptive pill (OCP) or HRT have an increased risk of thromboembolism.

Monitoring and follow-up

Postoperative pain

- Pain scores to ensure efficacy of analgesic regime
- Presence of adverse effects (e.g. sedation, constipation, nausea or vomiting) from opioids
- Respiratory rate if receiving opiates
- Ensure that patient is receiving the most appropriate analgesia – remember to step down as well as step up treatment according to the analgesic ladder

Postoperative nausea and vomiting

- Frequency of nausea and vomiting

Other postoperative complications

- Signs of infection (e.g. raised temperature, raised white cell count (WCC)/CRP)
- Signs of thromboembolism (e.g. swollen calves, shortness of breath)
- Ensure antibiotics are not continued unnecessarily and are converted to oral from IV when appropriate
- Review the need for prophylactic heparin when the patient is mobile

Outcomes of care

The patient will have:

- all of their usual medication prescribed
- postoperative complications (thromboembolism, infection) prevented
- postoperative pain, constipation, nausea and vomiting treated effectively
- minimal adverse effects from medication used to treat these problems

Table 2.12 Some subproblems seen in patients requiring surgery

Subproblem	Outcome of treatment	Assessment	Treatment options and implementation	Monitoring
SG1.1: Ensure usual medicines are prescribed where appropriate	• Patient's other medical conditions are managed effectively	• Medicines currently being taken by the patient • Type of surgery patient is to undergo	• See references on page 117	• As per condition being treated
SG1.2: Postoperative pain	• Control pain effectively • Minimise side-effects	• Type of pain being experienced • Severity of pain • Type of surgery undertaken	• Use analgesic ladder • No evidence tramadol is any better than other weak opioids • PCAs or epidurals may be needed	• Pain scores – review daily • Presence of side-effects
SG1.3: Postoperative nausea and vomiting	• Relieve nausea and vomiting	• Due to surgery? • Due to medication (e.g. analgesia) • Risk score	• Cyclizine or prochlorperazine is traditionally the first-line option • Ondansetron may be used in severe cases	• Frequency of nausea and vomiting
SG 1.4: Surgical site infection	• Prevent /treat surgical site infection	• Type of surgery • Previous allergies to antibiotics • Risk of endocarditis?	• Prophylactic antibiotics as per local policy	• Signs of infection (e.g. raised temperature, WCC, CRP)
SG1.5: Postoperative thromboembolism	• Prevent postoperative thromboembolic events	• Type of surgery • Period of immobility • Other risk factors (e.g. overweight, smoker) • Risk score as local policy	• Unfractionated heparin 5000 units 8–12-hourly • Low-dose LMWH (e.g. dalteparin 2500 or 5000 units daily depending on type of surgery)	• Signs of thromboembolism • Platelet counts if treatment longer than 5 days
SG 1.6: Constipation	• Relieve constipation without causing diarrhoea	• Due to immobility? • Due to medication? • Due to dehydration?	• Use stimulant and softener (e.g. senna and lactulose) • Keep well hydrated	• Stool frequency • Review before discharge
SG1.7: Fluid requirements	See **Surgical and general problems SG2**			

**Self-assessment questions:
Surgical and general 1** (Answers on p. 128)

1. It is necessary to stop certain medications up to several weeks before surgery. Give examples of such medicines and reasons for your answer.
2. Which of the following drugs should be discontinued during the perioperative period? Give reasons for your answers.
   • Prednisolone
   • Warfarin
   • Metformin
3. How may surgical site infections be prevented? Which types of surgery carry the highest risk of infection?
4. Why are patients who undergo surgery at risk of developing thromboembolism? How may this be prevented?
5. Do all surgical patients require thromboprophylaxis?
6. What advantages and disadvantages do low-molecular-weight heparins (LMWHs) have compared with unfractionated heparins in preventing thromboembolism?
7. How is a patient's pain assessed after surgery?
8. What methods are available for administering analgesia post-surgery?
9. What factors contribute to constipation in patients who undergo surgery? How should it be managed?

Surgical and general 2 problem: the patient requires intravenous fluids or nutrition

! Objectives of this section

The reader should be able to detail:
• the patients who require IV fluids
• the commonly used fluids available
• factors affecting the selection and modification of the fluid regime
• the dangers of using IV fluids incorrectly
• the patients who will require IV nutrition
• monitoring required to ensure efficacy and safety of IV therapy

Further reading: basics

• *British National Formulary*, current edn. London: Royal Pharmaceutical Society and British Medical Association. Sections 9.2.2: Parenteral preparations for fluid and electrolyte imbalance; and 9.3: Intravenous nutrition. (ONLINE)
• Murphy A, Scott A. Artificial nutritional support – what are the options? *Hosp Pharm* 2000; 7: 146–154. (ONLINE)
• National Institute for Health and Clinical Excellence. *Clinical Guideline 32: Nutrition Support in Adults*. London: NICE; 2006. (ONLINE)

Table 2.13 Available isotonic IV fluids

Fluid	Sodium	Potassium	Energy	Notes
5% glucose (dextrose) IV infusion	Nil	Nil	200 kcal/L	Also available ready mixed with potassium chloride, typically at 0.2% (27 mmmol/L) or 0.3% (40 mmol/L) suitable for peripheral infusion
0.9% sodium chloride IV infusion ('normal saline')	150 mmol/L	Nil	Nil	
Sodium lactate IV infusion ('Hartmann's', 'Ringer–lactate')	131 mmol/L	5 mmol/L	Nil	Contains 29 mmol bicarbonate/L as lactate – mostly used in surgery

Chart 2.22 Surgical and general 2 problem: the patient requires intravenous fluids or nutrition

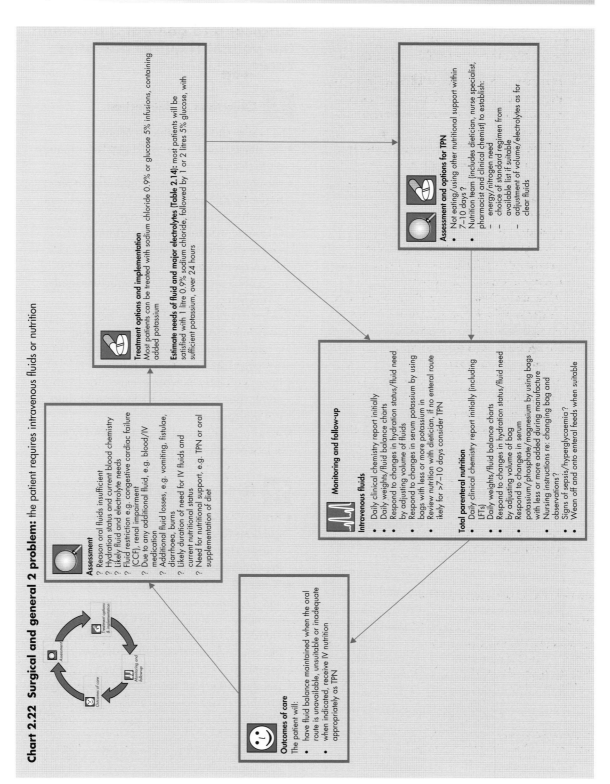

Assessment

- ? Reason oral fluids insufficient
- ? Hydration status and current blood chemistry
- ? Likely fluid and electrolyte needs
- ? Fluid restriction e.g. congestive cardiac failure (CCF), renal impairment
- ? Due to any additional fluid, e.g. blood/IV medication
- ? Additional fluid losses, e.g. vomiting, fistulae, diarrhoea, burns
- ? Likely duration of need for IV fluids and current nutritional status
- ? Need for nutritional support, e.g. TPN or oral supplementation of diet

Treatment options and implementation

Most patients can be treated with sodium chloride 0.9% or glucose 5% infusions, containing added potassium

Estimate needs of fluid and major electrolytes (Table 2.14): most patients will be satisfied with 1 litre 0.9% sodium chloride, followed by 1 or 2 litres 5% glucose, with sufficient potassium, over 24 hours

Assessment and options for TPN

- Not eating/using other nutritional support within 7–10 days?
- Nutrition team (includes dietician, nurse specialist, pharmacist and clinical chemist) to establish:
  - energy/nitrogen need
  - choice of standard regimen from available list if suitable
  - adjustment of volume/electrolytes as for clear fluids

Monitoring and follow-up

Intravenous fluids

- Daily clinical chemistry report initially
- Daily weights/fluid balance charts
- Respond to changes in hydration status/fluid need by adjusting volume of fluids
- Respond to changes in serum potassium by using bags with less or more potassium in
- Review nutrition with dietician, if no enteral route likely for >7–10 days consider TPN

Total parenteral nutrition

- Daily clinical chemistry report initially (including LFTs)
- Daily weights/fluid balance charts
- Respond to changes in hydration status/fluid need by adjusting volume of bag
- Respond to changes in serum potassium/phosphate/magnesium by using bags with less or more added during manufacture
- Nursing instructions re: changing bag and observations?
- Signs of sepsis/hyperglycaemia?
- Wean off and onto enteral feeds when suitable

Outcomes of care

The patient will:

- have fluid balance maintained when the oral route is unavailable, unsuitable or inadequate
- when indicated, receive IV nutrition appropriately as TPN

Table 2.14 Fluid and major electrolyte needs

Need	24-h need	Notes
Water	2–3 L/day	Best based on expected fluid output, plus 500 mL for 'insensible losses'. Avoid overload or dehydration
Sodium	2 mmol/kg	Adjusted against blood chemistry and atypical expected requirements
Potassium	1 mmol/kg	

SAQ Self-assessment questions:
Surgical and general 2
(Answers on p. 130)

1. Why might patients require IV fluid administration?
2. How is the volume of fluid required calculated?
3. What clear fluids are commonly used?
4. How are these solutions administered?
5. What are the possible dangers of clear fluid infusions?
6. If patients are receiving IV fluids for more than 24 hours, potassium is usually added to the bags. Why is this needed?
7. What are the dangers associated with IV administration of potassium, and how may these be prevented?
8. How long can a patient be maintained using IV fluids?
9. What is total parenteral nutrition (TPN)?
10. What are the contraindications to TPN?
11. How is TPN prescribed?
12. What are the possible complications of TPN?

Surgical and general 3 problem: the patient requires palliative care

 Objectives of this section

The reader should be able to detail:
- the objectives of care in patients who require palliative care
- the common problems encountered in patients requiring palliative care and their treatment:
  — pain – opioids, NSAIDs, tricyclic antidepressants, anticonvulsants
  — constipation – senna, lactulose, co-danthramer
  — nausea and vomiting – metoclopramide, cyclizine
  — restlessness and agitation – benzodiazepines
  — respiratory secretions – hyoscine hydrobromide
  — hallucinations – haloperidol
- the use of subcutaneous syringe drivers to administer medication when the oral route is not appropriate
- monitoring required to ensure efficacy and safety of drug therapy.

 Further reading: basics

- *British National Formulary*, current edn. London: Royal Pharmaceutical Society and British Medical Association. Introduction: Prescribing in palliative care. (ONLINE)
- Walker R, Edwards C, eds. *Clinical Pharmacy and Therapeutics*, 3rd edn. London: Churchill Livingstone; 2003. Chapter 31: Pain.
- Dodds LJ, ed. *Drugs in Use*, 3rd edn. London: Pharmaceutical Press; 2003. Chapter 22: Symptom control in palliative care.
- Randall MD, Neil KE. *Disease Management*. London: Pharmaceutical Press; 2004. Chapter 29: The cancer patient: cancer and palliative care.

Chart 2.23 Surgical and general 3 problem: the patient requires palliative care

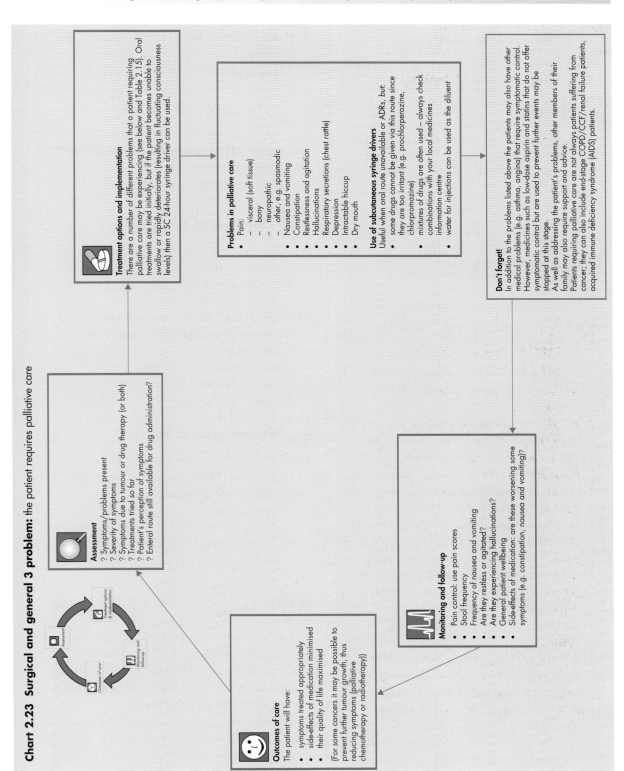

Assessment

? Symptoms/problems present
? Severity of symptoms
? Symptoms due to tumour or drug therapy (or both)
? Treatments tried so far
? Patient's perception of symptoms
? Enteral route still available for drug administration?

Treatment options and implementation

There are a number of different problems that a patient requiring palliative care may be experiencing (see below and Table 2.15). Oral treatments are tried initially, but if the patient becomes unable to swallow or rapidly deteriorates (resulting in fluctuating consciousness levels) then a SC 24-hour syringe driver can be used.

Problems in palliative care

- Pain:
  - visceral (soft tissue)
  - bony
  - neuropathic
  - other, e.g. spasmodic
- Nausea and vomiting
- Constipation
- Restlessness and agitation
- Hallucinations
- Respiratory secretions (chest rattle)
- Depression
- Intractable hiccup
- Dry mouth

Use of subcutaneous syringe drivers

Useful when oral route unavailable or ADRs, but:
- some drugs cannot be given via this route since they are too irritant (e.g. prochlorperazine, chlorpromazine)
- mixtures of drugs are often used – always check combinations with your local medicines information centre
- water for injections can be used as the diluent

Don't forget!

In addition to the problems listed above the patients may also have other medical problems (e.g. asthma, angina) that require symptomatic control. However, medicines such as low-dose aspirin and statins that do not offer symptomatic control but are used to prevent further events may be stopped at this stage.

As well as addressing the patient's problems, other members of their family may also require support and advice.

Patients requiring palliative care are not always patients suffering from cancer; they can also include end-stage COPD/CCF/renal failure patients, acquired immune deficiency syndrome (AIDS) patients.

Monitoring and follow-up

- Pain control: use pain scores
- Stool frequency
- Frequency of nausea and vomiting
- Are they restless or agitated?
- Are they experiencing hallucinations?
- General patient wellbeing
- Side-effects of medication: are these worsening some symptoms (e.g. constipation, nausea and vomiting)?

Outcomes of care

The patient will have:

- symptoms treated appropriately
- side-effects of medication minimised
- their quality of life maximised

(For some cancers it may be possible to prevent further tumour growth, thus reducing symptoms (palliative chemotherapy or radiotherapy))

Further reading: moving on

- Urie J, Fielding H, McArthur D, *et al.* Palliative care. *Pharm J* 2000; 265: 603–614. (ONLINE)

Guidelines

- Scottish Intercollegiate Guidelines Network. *SIGN 44: Control of Pain in Patients with Cancer.* Edinburgh: SIGN; 2000. (ONLINE)

SAQ **Self-assessment questions: Surgical and general 3**
(Answers on p. 132)

1. What questions should be asked when assessing a patient's pain control?
2. A patient requires morphine to be initiated for their pain. Discuss the different types of oral morphine preparations available and how they should be initiated.
3. A patient is receiving 120 mg bd of morphine sulphate SR tablets. What would be the required dose of morphine sulphate short-acting tablets/solution for breakthrough pain?
4. A patient has metastatic colon cancer and is thought to have bony metastases. The doctor increases the morphine sulphate SR tablet doses to help control the patient's pain. What would your response be?
5. A patient is prescribed morphine sulphate SR tablets for pain and is constipated. What would be the most appropriate laxative?
6. A patient is receiving morphine sulphate SR tablets 150 mg bd, morphine sulphate short-acting tablets 50 mg when required and co-danthramer 10 mL bd, and is now unable to take anything orally. What options exist for administration of these medicines by alternative routes? Include doses in your answer.

7. What issues need to be considered when commencing a patient on a subcutaneous syringe driver?

Surgical and general 4 problem: the patient has had a thromboembolic event

Objectives of this section

The reader should be able to detail:

- the objectives of care in patients who have either a deep vein thrombosis (DVT) or pulmonary embolism (PE)
- the risk factors for developing a DVT or PE
- the use and monitoring of heparin therapy
- the use and monitoring of oral anticoagualant (warfarin) therapy
- monitoring required to ensure efficacy and safety of drug therapy.

Further reading: basics

- *British National Formulary*, current edn. London: Royal Pharmaceutical Society and British Medical Association. Section 2.8: Anticoagulants and protamine. (ONLINE)
- Walker R, Edwards C, eds. *Clinical Pharmacy and Therapeutics*, 3rd edn. London: Churchill Livingstone; 2003. Chapters 31: Pain and 21: Thrombosis.

Guidelines

- Haemostasis and Thrombosis Task Force for the British Committee for Standards in Haematology. Guideline. Guidelines on oral anticoagulation: third edition. *Br J Haematol* 1998; 101: 374–387. (ONLINE)
- British Society of Haematology. *Guidelines on Oral Anticoagulation (Warfarin)*, 3rd edn, 2005 update. London: British Society of Haematology; 2005. (ONLINE)

Table 2.15 Some subproblems in patients requiring palliative care

Subproblem	Outcome of treatment	Assessment	Treatment options and implementation	Monitoring
SG3.1: Pain	• Maintain control of pain • Minimise side-effects of medication	• Type of pain patient has (e.g. visceral, bony, neuropathic) • Psychological factors present (e.g. depression, anxiety) which can worsen pain • Current severity of pain being experienced	• Visceral pain: use analgesic step ladder (start with regular paracetamol, then weak opioids, then strong opioids) • Bony pain: NSAIDs (no evidence that COX-2 inhibitors are any better), bisphosphonates (IV pamidronate) • Neuropathic pain: low-dose tricyclics (e.g. amitriptyline), anticonvulsants (carbamazepine, gabapentin), steroids (usually dexamethasone)	• Pain scores • Presence of ADRs
SG3.2: Constipation	• Maintain usual stool frequency • Relieve pain caused by constipation • Avoid diarrhoea	• Due to malignancy? • Due to medication? • Due to hypercalcaemia (from bone metastases)?	• If opioid induced use a stimulant plus a softener (co-danthramer offers the advantage of fewer tablets) • Enemas/suppositories if NBM	• Stool frequency
SG3.3: Nausea and vomiting	• Relieve or prevent nausea and vomiting	• Due to malignancy? • Due to medication? • Due to constipation? • Due to hypercalcaemia?	• Metoclopramide: may need up to 90 mg per day • Levomepromazine can be used for breakthrough nausea • If the patient has hypercalcaemia give IV bisphosphonate (pamidronate or zolendronate)	• Frequency of nausea or vomiting?
SG3.4: Restlessness and agitation	• Keep the patient settled • Avoid excessive sedation	• Severity of agitation	• Midazolam SC (unlicensed route but widely used)	• Is the patient settled? • Are they drowsy?
SG3.5: Hallucinations	• Avoid hallucinations	• Due to medication (e.g. opioids or steroids)? • Due to brain metastases?	• Haloperidol 1.5 mg nocte initially and titrate upwards) • Dexamethasone for brain metastases (not after 6 pm to avoid insomnia)	• Presence of hallucinations?

Table 2.15 Some subproblems in patients requiring palliative care *(continued)*

Subproblem	Outcome of treatment	Assessment	Treatment options and implementation	Monitoring
SG3.6: Respiratory secretions	• Reduce or prevent respiratory secretions	• Usually encountered in terminal phase	• Hyoscine hydrobromide • Glycopyrronium is less sedating and may be preferred if patient is already sedated	• Is the patient making a rattling sound? • Consciousness level
SG3.7: The patient is unable to take oral medication	• Ensure that patient receives as many of their medicines as possible	• Is medication essential? • Are alternative routes of administration available?	• Alternative routes: rectal, SC route is preferred to IM route as it is less painful for the patient	• See individual problems

**SAQ Self-assessment questions:
Surgical and general 4**

(Answers on p. 134)

1. What are the advantages of using LMWHs compared with unfractionated heparin for the initial management of a patient with a suspected DVT or PE?
2. What are the side-effects of long-term heparin use?
3. What time of day should patients be told to take their warfarin? What should they do if they forget to take it at this time?
4. If a patient who is pregnant developed a DVT, how should she be managed?
5. What would be the target INR and length of treatment for the following cases:
   • a patient with recurrent DVTs?
   • a patient receiving warfarin therapy for a PE who develops a second PE while receiving this treatment?
6. Why should warfarin therapy be avoided in patients who have recurrent falls or suffer with chronic confusion?
7. If a patient receiving warfarin therapy were to be commenced on the following medicines, what action should the pharmacist take
   • carbamazepine?
   • erythromycin?
   • atenolol?
8. A patient comes to your community pharmacy and requests St John's wort. After further questioning you discover that they are taking warfarin. What would be your response?

Chart 2.24 Surgical and general 4 problem: the patient has had a thromboembolic event

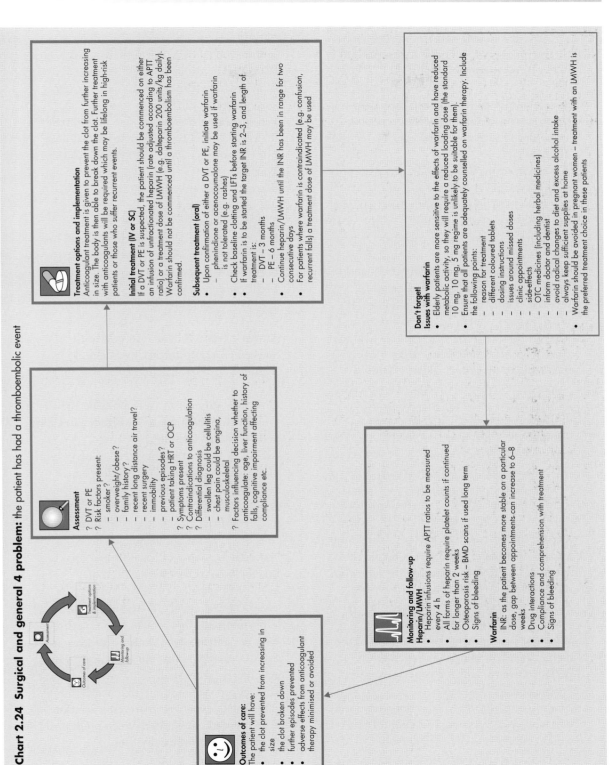

Assessment

? DVT or PE
? Risk factors present:
  – smoker ?
  – overweight/obese ?
  – family history ?
  – recent long distance air travel ?
  – recent surgery
  – immobility
  – previous episodes ?
  – patient taking HRT or OCP
? Symptoms present
? Contraindications to anticoagulation
? Differential diagnosis
  – swollen leg could be cellulitis
  – chest pain could be angina, musculoskeletal
? Factors influencing decision whether to anticoagulate: age, liver function, history of falls, cognitive impairment affecting compliance etc.

Treatment options and implementation

Anticoagulant treatment is given to prevent the clot from further increasing in size. The body is then able to break down the clot. Further treatment with anticoagulants will be required which may be lifelong in high-risk patients or those who suffer recurrent events.

Initial treatment (IV or SC)

If a DVT or PE is suspected, the patient should be commenced on either an infusion of unfractionated heparin (rate adjusted according to APTT ratio) or a treatment dose of LMWH (e.g. dalteparin 200 units/kg daily). Warfarin should not be commenced until a thromboembolism has been confirmed.

Subsequent treatment (oral)

- Upon confirmation of either a DVT or PE, initiate warfarin
  – phenindione or acenocoumalone may be used if warfarin is not tolerated (e.g. rashes)
- Check baseline clotting and LFTs before starting warfarin
- If warfarin is to be started the target INR is 2–3, and length of treatment is:
  – DVT – 3 months
  – PE – 6 months
- Continue heparin/LMWH until the INR has been in range for two consecutive days
- For patients where warfarin is contraindicated (e.g. confusion, recurrent falls) a treatment dose of LMWH may be used

Don't forget!

Issues with warfarin

- Elderly patients are more sensitive to the effects of warfarin and have reduced metabolic activity, so they will require a reduced loading dose (the standard 10 mg, 10 mg, 5 mg regime is unlikely to be suitable for them).
- Ensure that all patients are adequately counselled on warfarin therapy. Include the following points:
  – reason for treatment
  – different coloured tablets
  – dosing instructions
  – issues around missed doses
  – clinic appointments
  – side-effects
  – OTC medicines (including herbal medicines)
  – inform doctor and dentist
  – avoid radical changes to diet and excess alcohol intake
  – always keep sufficient supplies at home
- Warfarin should be avoided in pregnant women – treatment with an LMWH is the preferred treatment choice in these patients

Monitoring and follow-up

Heparin/LMWH

- Heparin infusions require APTT ratios to be measured every 4 h
- All forms of heparin require platelet counts if continued for longer than 2 weeks
- Osteoporosis risk – BMD scans if used long term
- Signs of bleeding

Warfarin

- INR: as the patient becomes more stable on a particular dose, gap between appointments can increase to 6–8 weeks
- Drug interactions
- Compliance and comprehension with treatment
- Signs of bleeding

Outcomes of care:

The patient will have:
- the clot prevented from increasing in size
- the clot broken down
- further episodes prevented
- adverse effects from anticoagulant therapy minimised or avoided

Answers to self-assessment questions:
Surgical and general 1: the patient is
to have surgery (p. 120)

1. **It is necessary to stop certain medications**
   up to several weeks before surgery. Give
   examples of such cases and reasons for your
   answer.
   Aspirin needs to be stopped 7–10 days prior
   to prostate and retinal surgery due to the
   associated risk of bleeding in these patients.
   For other groups of patients the risks versus
   the benefits of continuing treatment need to
   be considered.

   The oral contraceptive pill (OCP) and
   hormone replacement therapy (HRT)
   increase the risk of thromboembolism. If
   possible these should be stopped prior to
   surgery. If cessation is not possible (e.g. the
   patient requires emergency surgery or
   menopausal symptoms return if HRT is
   stopped) it is essential that patients receive
   adequate thromboprophylactic measures,
   e.g. heparin and graduated stockings.

   Tamoxifen also increases the risk of
   venous thromboembolism. The risks versus
   the benefits of continuing treatment need to
   be considered for each patient.

   MAOIs can have fatal interactions with
   anaesthetic drugs. Since MAOIs are usually
   a last resort for the treatment of depression,
   a safer anaesthetic technique is preferred to
   avoid having to stop these agents. However,
   if general anaesthesia is required, MAOIs
   should be discontinued two weeks before
   surgery.

2. **Which of the following drugs should be**
   discontinued during the perioperative
   period? Give reasons for your answers.
   Prednisolone
   This must be continued since long-term use
   will have resulted in adrenal suppression
   which will prevent the patient from
   mounting the necessary stress response

during surgery. If the patient is nil by
mouth, use IV hydrocortisone instead.
Patients will also require an additional dose
of IV hydrocortisone on the day of surgery,
since they will not be able to mount the
necessary stress response. The dose should
then be reduced to the patient's usual dose
postoperatively.
Warfarin
Warfarin should be temporarily
discontinued due to the risk of bleeding.
Patients should be converted to an IV
heparin infusion which can be reversed just
prior to surgery and restarted once the
operation is complete.
Metformin
Treatment should be discontinued while the
patient is 'nil-by-mouth' (NBM). If the
patient's blood glucose levels do not
markedly rise, no further treatment is
required. If blood glucose levels rise, IV
insulin will be required.

3. **How may surgical site infections be**
   prevented? Which types of surgery carry the
   highest risk of infection?
   Administration of prophylactic antibiotics at
   induction and for a couple of doses after
   surgery can reduce the risk of surgical site
   infection. Major abdominal surgery carries
   the highest risk of infection. In addition,
   consideration should be paid to the
   National Academy of Sciences National
   Research Council's classification of
   operations as being either 'clean',
   'clean-contaminated', 'contaminated' or
   'dirty-infected'.

4. **Why are patients who undergo surgery at**
   risk of developing thromboembolism? How
   may this be prevented?
   The period of immobility that a surgical
   patient may experience can result in stasis
   of the venous circulation, which predisposes
   a patient to thromboembolism.

   $\rightarrow$

Hypercoagulability of the blood can arise as a result of dehydration, acquired conditions (e.g. antiphospholipid syndromes), inherited conditions (e.g. factor V Leiden mutation) and the stress response mounted during surgery. Drugs, including HRT, the combined OCP and tamoxifen, can also predispose a patient to thromboembolism. The type of surgery involved also needs to be considered – major orthopaedic surgery carries the highest risk of thromboembolism. In addition, obesity and smoking are modifiable risk factors for thromboembolism and should be addressed before surgery. The prevention of thromboembolism involves prophylactic heparin, thromboembolic deterrent (TED) stockings and mobilising the patient as soon as possible.

5. **Do all surgical patients require thromboprophylaxis?**

This will depend on the type of surgery and other risk factors (see question 4) – each patient is given a risk assessment score. A patient undergoing a tonsillectomy is at a low risk of developing a thromboembolism since the surgery is minor and they are unlikely to be immobile for a significant period of time. However, a patient undergoing a hip replacement is at much greater risk due to the nature of the surgery and the long period of immobility that they will experience.

6. **What advantages and disadvantages do LMWHs have compared with unfractionated heparins in preventing thromboembolism?**

Prophylactic doses of both unfractionated heparins and LMWHs do not require monitoring of clotting times. LMWHs have the advantage that they can be given once daily, whereas unfractionated heparin needs to be given two or three times daily. LMWHs are also associated with a lower

risk of thrombocytopenia. LMWHs are more expensive and more difficult to reverse with protamine (if bleeding occurs) than unfractionated heparins.

7. **How is a patient's pain assessed after surgery?**

Pain scores are used to assess the severity of pain. One of the methods used involves asking the patient to give their pain a score out of 10, where 0 = no pain and 10 = worst pain they've ever had. Pain scores need to be assessed daily and analgesia adjusted to meet the patient's needs.

8. **What methods are available for administering analgesia post-surgery?**

Many patients will be able to tolerate oral medication post-surgery, thus this route should be tried wherever possible. If the oral route is not available a number of options exist:

- **IV/IM/SC doses on a when-required** basis – the disadvantage of this approach is that it relies on the patient experiencing pain before analgesia is administered, which is far from ideal.

- **Patient-controlled analgesia (PCA)** allows patients to titrate their own opioid dose, via an infusion pump, according to their needs. The patient receives a background infusion of opioid and can receive additional doses by pressing a button when required. Limits are set for both the dose received and the time interval between doses, to avoid excessive dosing.

- **Epidural analgesia:** a local anaesthetic such as bupivacaine is introduced into the space outside the dura. The addition of an opioid lowers the concentration of local anaesthetic required. This minimises leg muscle weakness, affording the patient greater

(Continued)

mobility. Epidurals may be patient controlled – the principles of PCA apply here too.

- **Suppositories:** paracetamol, NSAIDs and opioids are available as suppositories and may be appropriate if the patient has a needle phobia. If considering using the rectal route in a patient undergoing colorectal surgery, check that the patient has not had their rectum removed during surgery!

9. What factors contribute to constipation in patients who undergo surgery? How should it be managed?

Contributory factors include: patient immobility, opioid medication and dehydration. The use of stimulant laxatives (unless contraindicated) with softeners is the preferred option. In addition ensure that the patient is well hydrated and they mobilise as soon as possible, and reduce opioid use where possible.

 Answers to self-assessment questions:
Surgical and general 2: intravenous fluids or nutrition (p. 122)

1. Why might patients require IV fluid administration?

Patients who cannot maintain adequate hydration by mouth require clear 'crystalloid' fluids to maintain organ perfusion and function, and homeostasis. The patients may be NBM due to surgery or their medical condition, or simply be experiencing vomiting or diarrhoea. In other patients, fluids are required to administer drug therapy such as aminophylline or antibiotics intravenously or to correct a severe dehydration or hypotension.

2. How is the volume of fluid required calculated?

Exact precision is not necessary in most patients. A range of formulae of varying complexity is used but empirical principles usually suffice – most patients need 2–3 L daily. Small frail old patients need less, as fluid overload (with pulmonary oedema) can occur due to cardiac and renal impairment, and younger, fitter patients need more. If a patient is initially overloaded, less fluid should be

administered and, conversely, initial dehydration, losses in surgical drains, diarrhoea and vomiting will increase requirements. Insensible losses (respiration, sweat, metabolic processes, faeces etc.) should not be forgotten – they can amount to substantial volumes.

3. What clear fluids are commonly used?

Sodium chloride 0.9% ('normal saline') and glucose 5% (dextrose) are the two most commonly used IV fluids. A litre of sodium chloride provides 150 millimoles of sodium, approximately the normal daily need, and any extra fluid can be provided with 5% dextrose, which is effectively just water. Mixed solutions exist but offer few advantages in most patients – as with many things in pharmacy the simplest solutions are safest and easiest to prescribe and administer.

4. How are these solutions administered?

Each bag can be administered sequentially. If a patient is receiving 3 litres daily, this would be 1 litre every 8 hours, which is 125 mL/h. A pump is not always necessary but prevents over-/under-infusion, particularly safe when potassium-containing solutions are being infused.

$\longrightarrow$

5. **What are the possible dangers of clear fluid infusions?**

If too much fluid is instilled into a patient without the renal capacity to excrete it, it will accumulate and fluid overload can develop. Daily weights and fluid-balance measurements, where inputs and outputs are recorded, will establish the ongoing need. If a patient is to receive, for example, blood transfusions, the volume to be infused should be taken into account.

6. **If patients are receiving IV fluids for more than 24 hours, potassium is usually added to the bags. Why is this needed?**

If the patient is not taking anything orally, their potassium intake will be zero. If IV fluids are given, this will dilute the patient's serum potassium, which may result in cardiac arrhythmias and muscle weakness.

7. **What are the dangers associated with IV administration of potassium, and how may these be prevented?**

Intravenous potassium can be deadly if not used properly. If concentrated potassium is administered as a bolus it can cause fatal cardiac arrhythmias (there have been numerous reported cases of this). In addition, IV potassium is irritant and can result in thrombophlebitis if the infusion is given at too high a concentration in a peripheral vein. When potassium is added to infusion fluids it can produce a layering effect if it is not mixed adequately (resulting in the formation of 'pockets' of potassium).

To eliminate errors with concentrated potassium, many hospitals have removed ampoules of potassium chloride from wards and purchase ready-mixed bags. Hospitals should also have policies in place that advise medical staff on the maximum concentration of potassium that can be administered peripherally (40 mmoles in 500 mL is considered the maximum concentration that can be given peripherally).

8. **How long can a patient be maintained using IV fluids?**

There is no formal limit, although the infusion site will need rotating every few days. However, although sodium, potassium and water needs are being met, there is a complete inadequacy of calories, and no protein, vitamins or trace elements. The patient is effectively starving and this will affect healing and recovery if feeding is not restarted. Feeding through nasogastric or percutaneous endoscopic gastrostomy tubes (PEGs) may be needed, but if no enteral route is available then TPN will be needed after 7–10 days. If it is known in advance that enteral nutrition will not be restored within that time frame, TPN should be prescribed immediately.

9. **What is TPN?**

Put simply, TPN is a complete diet infused, usually through a large 'central' vein, from a single aseptically prepared 'all-in-one' bag over 24 hours. It contains all the fluid, electrolytes, protein (as amino acids), fat (as lipid emulsions), carbohydrate (as glucose), fat-soluble and water-soluble vitamins, and trace elements that the patient needs. Patients can thrive on TPN for many years.

10. **What are the contraindications to TPN?**

If the patient is in the terminal phase of an illness, then TPN is considered unethical. However, although a functioning gut was formerly considered a contraindication to TPN therapy, increasingly patients are receiving IV nutrition as a support to other means of feeding.

11. **How is TPN prescribed?**

A range of standard mixtures is defined in hospitals or by the ingredients' manufacturers, to provide a determined energy/nitrogen load in a fixed volume.

(Continued)

Most patients can be fed perfectly well on one of a small number of the standard mixtures. Based on the blood tests that will be required frequently at first, electrolytes can be adjusted on a daily basis at the manufacturing stage.

12. **What are the possible complications of TPN?**
As with clear fluids, fluid overload and electrolyte imbalances are possible if the patient is not monitored properly or the results of that monitoring are not acted upon. Hyperglycaemia from the infusion of hypertonic dextrose into stressed patients may require insulin support. However, the biggest danger is septicaemia. Patients should have their infusions changed under conditions of the strictest asepsis – one of the advantages of the 'all-in-one' bag is that the infusion line should be getting broken only once a day. Patients should be monitored for fever or redness at the infusion site, and any sepsis treated aggressively by removing the line and prescribing IV antibiotics in line with local policies. Derangements in liver function tests may respond to a change in the lipid used in the TPN bag.

 Answers to self-assessment questions: Surgical and general 3: palliative care (p. 124)

1. **What questions should be asked when assessing a patient's pain control?**
In order to assess a patient's pain control, the following questions should be asked:
   - Where is the pain located?
   - What type(s) of pain does the patient have? The nature of the patient's pain may be visceral (soft tissue), bony (due to metastases) or neuropathic. These different types of pain respond to different groups of analgesics
   - How severe is the pain?
   - Which analgesics have been tried so far and what effect have they had on the patient's pain?
   - Is the patient depressed? Depression and anxiety can worsen a patient's pain.

2. **A patient requires morphine to be initiated for their pain. Discuss the different types of oral morphine preparations available and how they should be initiated.**

- **Short-acting preparations (available as tablets and liquid):** these need to be given frequently and are usually started at a dose of 10–20 mg every 4 hours, with the same dose being prescribed 'prn' for breakthrough pain. Patients who are elderly or have hepatic or renal impairment will require a lower initial dose. The dose is reviewed every few days, taking into account the number of 'prn' doses required by the patient. The problem with this approach is that on busy wards patients may not receive their doses regularly and start to worry – which can worsen their pain.
- **Long-acting preparations (available as once or twice daily SR tablets/capsules):** once a patient is stabilised on an appropriate dose of short-acting morphine they can be converted to a long-acting preparation to allow for less frequent dosing and minimisation of side-effects (by flattening the peak serum concentrations). The usual starting dose

$\rightarrow$

would be 10–30 mg bd (depending on previous exposure to opioids) with short-acting morphine prescribed for breakthrough pain. The dose is readjusted every few days according to the number of doses of short-acting morphine prescribed.

3. **A patient is receiving 120 mg bd of morphine sulphate SR tablets. What would be the required dose of morphine sulphate short-acting tablets/solution for breakthrough pain?**

The patient is receiving 240 mg of morphine per day. The dose given for breakthrough pain is one-sixth of the total daily morphine dose. Thus 240 mg ÷ 6 = 40 mg for breakthrough pain.

4. **A patient has metastatic colon cancer and is thought to have bony metastases. The doctor increases the morphine sulphate SR tablet doses to help control the patient's pain. What would your response be?**

Opioids are not effective for bony pain. The most effective options are NSAIDs (there is no evidence that COX-2 inhibitors are any better than traditional NSAIDs) or IV bisphosphonates (pamidronate or zolendronate) which reduce bone resorption (breakdown).

5. **A patient is prescribed morphine sulphate SR tablets for pain and is constipated. What would be the most appropriate laxative?**

Since opiates reduce bowel motility, a stimulant laxative such as senna is required. A softener such as lactulose is often given in addition to allow easier passage of stools and reduce bowel spasms. Co-danthramer is often used in palliative care since it contains a stimulant and a softener. This treatment is licensed for use only in terminally ill patients owing to the possible

carcinogenicity associated with danthron.

6. **A patient is receiving morphine sulphate SR tablets 150 mg bd, morphine sulphate short-acting tablets/solution 50 mg when required and co-danthramer 10 mL bd, and is now unable to take anything orally. What options exist for administration of these medicines by alternative routes? Include doses in your answer.**

The oral morphine could be converted to either a fentanyl patch or a subcutaneous infusion of diamorphine. To convert to a fentanyl patch, 90 mg oral morphine is approximately equal to 25 micrograms/hour fentanyl patch. Thus a 75 microgram patch would be required for this patient.

The dose of subcutaneous diamorphine = one-third of the total daily morphine dose. Thus, the patient would require 100 mg SC over 24 hours. The dose of diamorphine required for breakthrough pain in both cases would be 15 mg.

The rectal route could be considered for administration of laxatives. To treat constipation bisacodyl suppositories, glycerine suppositories or enemas could be used.

7. **What issues need to be considered when commencing a patient on a subcutaneous syringe driver?**

The main issues to consider are: the drugs to be used, compatibility of drugs in solution, doses of drugs and volume of driver (to determine concentration of drugs in solution). Most medicines information centres will have access to information regarding the stability of mixtures of drugs in solution. For mixtures of drugs where no stability data exist, advise the nursing staff to inspect the syringe regularly for signs of precipitation.

Answers to self-assessment questions:
Surgical and general 4:
thromboembolic episode (p. 126)

1. **What are the advantages of using LMWHs compared with unfractionated heparin for the initial management of a patient with a suspected DVT or PE?**
Treatment doses of unfractionated heparins require regular monitoring of activated partial thromboplastin time (APTT) to calculate the APTT ratio, which is used to adjust the infusion rate. This is labour intensive for nursing staff. LMWH therapy does not require monitoring of APTT and is administered as a once-daily subcutaneous injection, reducing nursing time. LMWHs have also been shown to have a lower incidence of thrombocytopenia than unfractionated heparins. However, when considering drug costs alone, LMWHs are more expensive than unfractionated heparin.

2. **What are the side-effects of long-term heparin use?**
Recognised side-effects with sustained heparin use are bleeding, thrombocytopenia and osteoporosis.

3. **What time of day should patients take their warfarin? What should they do if they forget to take it at this time?**
Patients are usually told to take their warfarin at 6 pm. This allows them to have their INR measured in the morning and the corresponding evening's dose adjusted in light of this result if necessary. If they forget to take their warfarin at 6 pm, but remember before bedtime, it is alright to take it at that time. However, if they don't realise that they've missed their 6 pm dose until the next morning, they should be instructed to omit that dose and not to

double-up when taking that evening's dose. Missed doses should always be noted so that the anticoagulant clinic can take this into consideration and avoid unnecessary dose increases when the patient is next reviewed.

4. **If a patient who is pregnant developed a DVT, how should she be managed?**
Warfarin should be avoided during pregnancy since it has been shown to cross the placenta and cause fetal and neonatal haemorrhage as well as congenital malformations. Pregnant women who develop a thromboembolism should be prescribed LMWH treatment instead.

5. **What would be the target INR and length of treatment for the following cases:**
   • a patient with recurrent DVTs – INR range = 2–3, treatment would be lifelong
   • a patient receiving warfarin therapy for a PE who develops a second PE while receiving this treatment – INR range = 3–4, treatment would be for 6 months.

6. **Why should warfarin therapy be avoided in patients who have recurrent falls or suffer with chronic confusion?**
Patients who have recurrent falls are at risk of internal bleeding, which is worsened by warfarin therapy. Patients who are chronically confused are less likely to take their prescribed dose of warfarin properly; there is significant potential for the patient to both under- and overdose on warfarin therapy.

7. **If a patient who was stabilised on warfarin therapy was to be commenced on the following medicines, what action should the pharmacist take?**
   • **Carbamazepine**: carbamazepine induces cytochrome P450 enzymes, which can accelerate the metabolism of warfarin and

→

significantly reduce the INR. The INR should be monitored closely and the warfarin dose increased accordingly.

- **Erythromycin:** erythromycin is an inhibitor of cytochrome P450 enzymes, which can reduce the metabolism of warfarin and significantly increase a patient's INR. The INR should be monitored closely during therapy and for a few days after the course has finished, with dose adjustments made as appropriate
- **Atenolol:** there is no known interaction between warfarin and atenolol so the pharmacist is required to take no further action.

8. **A patient comes to your community pharmacy and requests St John's wort. After further questioning you discover that they are taking warfarin. What would be your response?**

The patient should be advised against purchasing St John's wort since it is an enzyme inducer, which has the potential to reduce a patient's INR. They should be referred to their GP if they are suffering from depression.

P Pharmaceutical problems

Introduction

Although most pharmaceutical care involves dealing with problems that would be recognised as such by doctors, pharmacists should think broadly and identify other problems that may give rise to morbidity and even mortality, and that are often overlooked.

 Problem 1: the patient has had a suspected adverse drug reaction (ADR)

Adverse events are common, especially in patients on multiple drug therapy, who usually have several medical problems and are often elderly. Patients may well have altered drug handling due to renal and hepatic impairment, and less functional reserve in many organ systems.

 Problem 2: the patient is receiving a drug with a narrow therapeutic index

Pharmacokinetics does not always involve calculations or the measurement of drug concentrations in body fluids. It does involve some consideration of how an individual patient might be handling drugs. Two practical examples (theophylline and phenytoin) demonstrate how pharmacists can assist in therapy.

 Problem 3: the patient has difficulties with compliance

Patients may not adhere to their prescribed drug regimes for a variety of reasons, many of which are understandable. Many chronic conditions require patients to take medication that may not make them feel any better, especially in the short term. For patients to receive full benefit from their therapies, compliance is important, however, and pharmacists can act to identify the reasons for non-compliance and provide appropriate advice.

 Problem 4: the patient's medication history is not easily identified

The role of the pharmacist in obtaining a drug history was discussed in Section 1 as part of the derivation of the problem list. However, what the patient has in reality been taking is often difficult to ascertain in the admission process or primary care interview, and the inadequacy of medication records can be a problem in itself.

 ## Problem 5: the patient is about to be discharged from hospital

When a patient is discharged from hospital back into their home environment, a transfer of care and responsibilities takes place that, if not handled appropriately, especially in vulnerable people, may lead to a speedy re-admission to hospital.

The pharmacist's role

Pharmaceutical care provides pharmacists with the opportunity to display skills that cannot be effectively duplicated by other professions. While there are many examples of excellent practice in the UK, services such as counselling, drug history taking and discharge planning are still not universally provided across the NHS. Properly applied, these services have the potential to make a real difference to patients' lives and prevent problems arising that may impair the achievement of the desired therapeutic outcome in many conditions.

Pharmaceutical 1 problem: the patient has had a suspected ADR

 ### Objectives of this section

The reader should be able to detail:
- the patients most at risk of ADRs
- the types of drugs most likely to cause ADRs
- mechanisms for pharmacovigilance.

 ### Further reading: basics

- Randall MD, Neil KE. *Disease Management*. London: Pharmaceutical Press; 2004.

Chapter 5: Adverse drug reactions and interactions.
- Walker R, Edwards C, eds. *Clinical Pharmacy and Therapeutics*, 3rd edn. London: Churchill Livingstone; 2003. Chapter 3: Adverse drug reactions.
- CSM Mersey. The burden of adverse drug reactions (ADRs). *Mersey ADR Newsletter 25.* Liverpool: CSM Mersey; 2005. (ONLINE)
- Cox A. Yellow card reporting scheme: what to report and where to. *Tomorrow's Pharmacist* 2005; 66–67. (ONLINE)

 ### Further reading: moving on

- Pirmohamed M, James S, Meakin S *et al.* Adverse drug reactions as cause of admission to hospital: prospective analysis of 18 820 patients. *BMJ* 2004; 329: 15–19. (ONLINE)
- Ferner R, Pirmohamed M. Monitoring drug treatment. *BMJ* 2003; 327: 1179–1181. (ONLINE)
- Pirmohamed M, Breckenridge AM, Kitteringham NR, Park BK. Fortnightly review: Adverse drug reactions. *BMJ* 1998; 316: 1295–1298. (ONLINE)
- Anon. International drug monitoring: the role of the hospital. A WHO report. *Drug Intell Clin Pharm* 1970; 4: 101–110.

 ### Guidelines

- Medicines and Healthcare Products Regulatory Agency/Committee on Safety of Medicines website. *The Yellow Card Scheme.* (ONLINE)

 SAQ Self-assessment questions: **Pharmaceutical 1**
(Answers on p. 149)

1. What is the definition of an ADR?
2. Why are ADRs a problem?
3. What is the incidence of ADRs?

(Questions continued on page 139)

Chart 2.25 Pharmaceutical 1 problem: the patient has a suspected adverse drug reaction

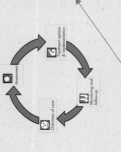

Assessment: higher-risk patients

- Patients with a history of ADRs/allergies
- Other pathologies
- Hepatic/renal/thyroid disorders/infectious diseases
- Patients with polypharmacy:
  - neonates/infants/elderly patients
  - patients taking therapy requiring monitoring; e.g. clozapine or DMARDs

Identification of ADRs

- Experience of the drugs in question can be useful
- Timing of the reaction in relation to when medication was administered or initiated
- Drug history: what has the patient taken in the last few weeks?
- Dechallenge: what happened when the drug was stopped?
- Rechallenge: what happened when the drug was restarted?
- Alternative causes: placebo effect, excipients, coincidence?
- Patient's concurrent disease states

Treatment options and implementation

- Consider 'risk:benefit' ratio: what are the risks of stopping therapy against continuing with the medication? For example, a minor side-effect would not result in stopping a life-saving therapy
- For type B reactions, stopping the drug would be necessary, but, for type A reactions, a reduction in dose may be appropriate
- Alterations to the timing of dose might be useful, to coincide with meals if a drug causes gastric irritation, or sleep if a drug causes drowsiness
- It is also possible to see if a drug's adverse effects wear off over time, e.g. nausea with morphine
- Finally, it is possible to manage ADRs with 'antidotes', e.g. procyclidine may treat the dystonic effects of antipsychotic therapy

Report to the CSM

For 'established' drugs, report:
- unusual or unexpected ADRs
- serious ADRs (fatal or life threatening, disabling or those that prolong or result in hospitalisation)

For 'black triangle' drugs report:
- any ADRs

Remember: 100% certainty of causality is not required to report an ADR to the MHRA/CSM, and you can report more than one drug as being the possible cause of a reaction.

Don't forget!

Make sure that any ADRs experienced by a patient are carefully documented in their medical records and in a visible place on their prescription chart. This will help avoid accidental re-exposure to the same drug.
There are also cases where cross-sensitivity exists within the same group of drugs, e.g. penicillins or antithyroid drugs, and this should also be considered.

Monitoring and follow-up

All drugs have some risk but those commonly associated with ADRs include:
- narrow therapeutic index/non-linear kinetics
- potential for interaction
- drugs with clinically important adverse effects:
  - antirheumatic drugs
  - immunosuppressants
  - cytotoxic drugs
  - NSAIDs
  - diuretics
  - corticosteroids
  - antithyroid drugs
  - cardiac glycosides

NB: this is not an exhaustive list.

Outcomes of care

The patient will have:
- a resolution of their ADR, where possible or appropriate
- appropriate documentation of their ADR
- their ADR reported to the CSM/MHRA where appropriate
- an alternative source of therapy, if appropriate
- their risk status assessed to minimise the potential for further ADRs

Self-assessment questions: Pharmaceutical 1

(Continued)

4. Should drugs that aren't safe be prevented from being marketed?
5. What is the difference between type A and type B reactions?
6. Which groups of drugs are most commonly associated with ADRs?
7. Why are elderly people at increased risk of experiencing an ADR?
8. Why is it difficult to detect ADRs?
9. What are the purposes of post-marketing surveillance?
10. For what reasons do healthcare professionals often fail to report ADRs?
11. What can the Medicines and Healthcare Products Regulatory Agency (MHRA) do about ADRs?
12. What are the limitations of Committee on Safety of Medicines (CSM) data?
13. What are the responsibilities of the pharmacist with regard to ADRs?

Pharmaceutical 2 problem: the patient is receiving a drug with a narrow therapeutic index

The assistance of Neil A Caldwell, MSc MRPharmS, Assistant Director of Pharmacy (Clinical Services), at Wirral Hospitals NHS Trust and Honorary Lecturer, Liverpool John Moores University, is gratefully acknowledged in the preparation of this section.

 Objectives of this section

The reader should be able to:
- apply clinical pharmacokinetics to patient care
- interpret blood concentrations of medicines in the light of other information available
- individualise therapy for patient care
- identify when blood concentrations require monitoring
- identify why blood concentrations of medicines are not always interpretable or necessary.

 Further reading: basics

- Randall MD, Neil KE. *Disease Management.* London: Pharmaceutical Press; 2004. Chapter 6: Clinical pharmacokinetics and therapeutic drug monitoring.
- Thomson A. Back to basics: pharmacokinetics. *Pharm J* 2004; 272: 769–771. (ONLINE)

 Further reading: moving on

- Thomson A. Why do therapeutic drug monitoring? *Pharm J* 2004; 272: 153–155. (ONLINE)
- Thomson A. Variability in drug dosage requirements. *Pharm J* 2004; 272: 806–808. (ONLINE)
- Thomson A. Examples of dosage regimen design. *Pharm J* 2004; 273: 188–190. (ONLINE)

 Assessing the patient

Pharmacokinetics describes the absorption, distribution, metabolism and excretion of drugs. It is a subject that is sometimes avoided by both students and practitioners. Many practitioners do not believe that it is relevant and that it always involves complex calculations. The aim of this chapter is to dispel this myth and show that many of you have been applying clinical pharmacokinetics to solve problems without realising it. It has been said, 'Pharmacokinetics is not a rare art, but an essential tool for providing patient care'.[1]

When dealing with any problem that requires the application of clinical pharmacokinetic methods (as with any other medicines information problem), it is vital that relevant information about the patient be gathered. Wrong advice may be given because inappropriate assumptions have been made. By considering the following points, such errors may be avoided.

1. **Is this appropriate drug treatment for the individual?** There is no point in wasting time calculating a dose if the wrong drug has been selected.

2. **Where is the drug absorbed and which factors affect absorption?** Absorption of tetracycline is impaired by calcium-containing products – thus patients should be advised to leave 2 hours either side of their tetracycline dose before consuming dairy products. Patients with short bowel syndrome may have rapid gastric transit and require administration of medicines by routes other than per oral. Patients suffering from small bowel Crohn's disease will have impaired absorption of vitamin B_{12} and thus require IM injections.

3. **How is the drug distributed in the body?** Is the drug water or fat soluble? Does it bind to plasma proteins? The volume of distribution of water-soluble drugs (e.g. gentamicin) will be increased in oedematous patients. In patients with a low serum albumin, the concentration of 'free' phenytoin will be increased, resulting in enhanced clinical effect relative to the reported total drug concentration.

4. **How is the drug eliminated?** This not only includes whether the drug is excreted unchanged in the urine or undergoes hepatic metabolism, but also requires a consideration of whether the metabolic products are pharmacologically active, toxic or inactive. For example, morphine has metabolites that are pharmacologically active.

5. **Are there any individual factors that may alter the clearance of the drug?** As well as considering the presence of renal or hepatic impairment, patients may be prescribed other drugs that alter the metabolism or elimination of the drug in question.

6. **Which order pharmacokinetics does the drug exhibit?** Most drugs exhibit first-order pharmacokinetics, where doubling the dose will double the drug concentration. However, phenytoin exhibits zero-order elimination and a relatively small increase in dose, when enzymatic capacity has become saturated, will produce a large increase in plasma concentration.

7. **If serum concentrations have been taken:**
   - **why have they been requested?** Will the reported concentration alter the treatment plan or has the management plan already been concluded? There are occasions when concentrations have been requested simply because they can be measured.
   - **were they taken at the right time?** If samples are taken at the wrong time they are much more difficult to interpret. Digoxin concentrations should be taken at least 6 hours after oral dosing to allow for distribution into the tissues – blood samples taken earlier result in falsely high concentrations.
   - **has there been laboratory error in processing the sample?** If concentrations inexplicably change despite no apparent change in dose it is worth considering whether the sample has been contaminated or an analytical error has occurred.
   - **is the patient at steady state?** It takes approximately five half-lives to reach steady state. If concentrations are taken before this time, the plasma concentrations of newly commenced therapies will continue to increase until steady state. Concentrations taken before steady state are more difficult to interpret but they are still useful to detect early drug toxicity and assess the appropriateness of loading doses.

8. **In addition to the pharmacokinetic differences between patient groups, consider also pharmacodynamic effects.** Elderly patients are more sensitive to the effects of sedatives and antihypertensives; patients with Addison's disease are more at risk of adrenal suppression if given corticosteroids for inflammatory conditions.

9. **How has the patient responded clinically?** If a patient receiving digoxin for fast atrial fibrillation has a plasma concentration of

0.8 micrograms/L (range 1–2 micrograms/L), but their pulse has fallen to 80 beats/minute, is an increase in dose required? It is important to remember that the published reference ranges for plasma concentrations are only a guide: treat the patient, not the plasma concentration.

Reference

1 Caldwell NA, Sexton J, Green CF. Pharmacokinetics is not a rare art but an essential tool for providing proper care. *Pharm J* 2001; 267: 50. (ONLINE)

Figure 2.1 What to do when a drug concentration is reported

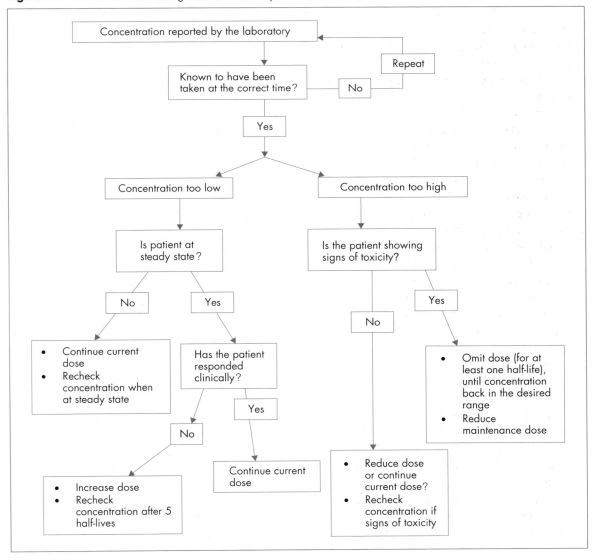

Chart 2.26 Pharmaceutical 2.1 problem: the patient is to be commenced on an aminophylline infusion

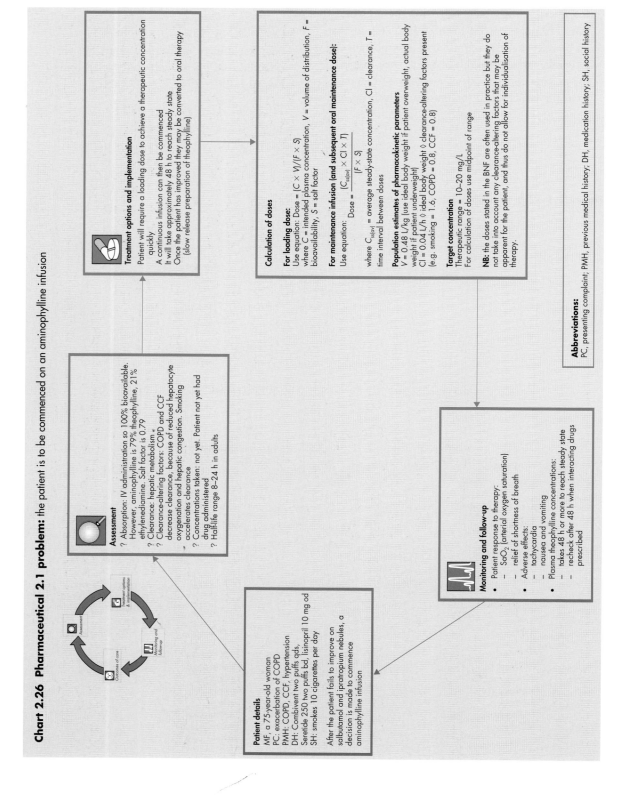

Patient details

MF, a 75-year-old woman

PC: exacerbation of COPD

PMH: COPD, CCF, hypertension

DH: Combivent two puffs qds,
Seretide 250 two puffs bd, lisinopril 10 mg od

SH: smokes 10 cigarettes per day

After the patient fails to improve on
salbutamol and ipratropium nebules, a
decision is made to commence an
aminophylline infusion

Assessment

? Absorption: IV administration so 100% bioavailable.
However, aminophylline is 79% theophylline, 21%
ethylenediamine. Salt factor is 0.79

? Clearance: hepatic metabolism

? Clearance-altering factors: COPD and CCF
decrease clearance, because of reduced hepatocyte
oxygenation and hepatic congestion. Smoking
accelerates clearance

? Concentrations taken: not yet. Patient not yet had
drug administered

? Half-life range 8–24 h in adults

Treatment options and implementation

Patient will require a loading dose to achieve a therapeutic concentration
quickly

A continuous infusion can then be commenced

It will take approximately 48 h to reach steady state

Once the patient has improved they may be converted to oral therapy
(slow release preparation of theophylline)

Calculation of doses

For loading dose:

Use equation: Dose = $(C \times V)/(F \times S)$

where C = intended plasma concentration, V = volume of distribution, F =
bioavailability, S = salt factor

For maintenance infusion (and subsequent oral maintenance dose):

Use equation: $\text{Dose} = \dfrac{(C_{\text{ss(av)}} \times Cl \times T)}{(F \times S)}$

where $C_{\text{ss(av)}}$ = average steady-state concentration, Cl = clearance, T =
time interval between doses

Population estimates of pharmacokinetic parameters

V = 0.48 L/kg (use ideal body weight if patient overweight, actual body
weight if patient underweight)

Cl = 0.04 L/h ◊ ideal body weight ◊ clearance-altering factors present
(e.g. smoking = 1.6, COPD = 0.8, CCF = 0.8)

Target concentration

Therapeutic range = 10–20 mg/L
For calculation of doses use midpoint of range

NB: the doses stated in the BNF are often used in practice but they do
not take into account any clearance-altering factors that may be
apparent for the patient, and thus do not allow for individualisation of
therapy.

Monitoring and follow-up

- Patient response to therapy:
  - SaO_2 (arterial oxygen saturation)
  - relief of shortness of breath
- Adverse effects:
  - tachycardia
  - nausea and vomiting
- Plasma theophylline concentrations:
  - takes 48 h or more to reach steady state
  - recheck after 48 h when interacting drugs
    prescribed

Abbreviations:

PC, presenting complaint; PMH, previous medical history; DH, medication history; SH, social history

Chart 2.27 Pharmaceutical 2.2 problem: the patient is experiencing phenytoin toxicity

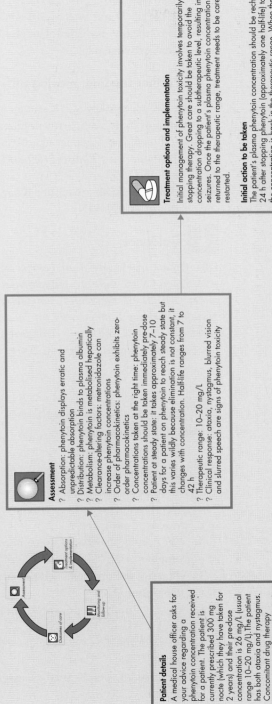

Patient details

A medical house officer asks for your advice regarding a phenytoin concentration received for a patient. The patient is currently prescribed 300 mg nocte (which they have taken for 2 years) and their pre-dose concentration is 26 mg/L (usual range 10–20 mg/L). The patient has both ataxia and nystagmus. Concomitant drug therapy consists of amlodipine 5 mg od and metronidazole 400 mg tds. Other blood tests are normal.

Assessment

? Absorption: phenytoin displays erratic and unpredictable absorption
? Distribution: phenytoin binds to plasma albumin
? Metabolism: phenytoin is metabolised hepatically
? Clearance-altering factors: metronidazole can increase phenytoin concentrations
? Order of pharmacokinetics: phenytoin exhibits zero-order pharmacokinetics
? Concentrations taken at the right time: phenytoin concentrations should be taken immediately pre-dose
? Patient at steady state: it takes approximately 7–10 days for a patient on phenytoin to reach steady state but this varies wildly because elimination is not constant, it changes with concentration. Half-life ranges from 7 to 42 h
? Therapeutic range: 10–20 mg/L
? Clinical response: ataxia, nystagmus, blurred vision and slurred speech are signs of phenytoin toxicity

Treatment options and implementation

Initial management of phenytoin toxicity involves temporarily stopping therapy. Great care should be taken to avoid the concentration dropping to a subtherapeutic level, resulting in seizures. Once the patient's plasma phenytoin concentration has returned to the therapeutic range, treatment needs to be carefully restarted.

Initial action to be taken

The patient's plasma phenytoin concentration should be rechecked 24 h after stopping phenytoin (approximately one half-life) to see if the concentration is back in the therapeutic range. When the patient's plasma concentration is in the desired range, the phenytoin may be restarted. It is possible that the metronidazole therapy is responsible for this increase in concentration.

Restarting phenytoin

If metronidazole needs to be continued then a reduction in phenytoin dose is needed – restart at 275 mg nocte and recheck concentrations 4–5 days later to ensure that the patient's concentration is not above the upper limit. A slight dose decrease is suggested because of the concentration-dependent elimination. Dose increases (to titrate back to the patient's original dose) may be considered only when the patient has reached steady state (after approximately 7–10 days) at a particular dose, and concentrations are not above the upper limit.
Once the course of metronidazole has finished, the phenytoin dose will need to be increased back to the previous dose (300 mg) and concentrations rechecked.

Monitoring and follow-up

- Seizure control
- Signs of toxicity:
  - monitor for ataxia and nystagmus and counsel patient to report these to doctor
- Plasma phenytoin concentrations:
  - recheck 4–5 days after resuming therapy to ensure that patient has not returned to toxic concentrations
- Serum albumin levels

Self-assessment questions:
Pharmaceutical 2

(Answers on p. 151)

1. Do all drugs for which plasma concentrations can be obtained require concentrations to be measured?
2. Give some justifiable reasons for requesting a drug concentration measurement to be obtained from a patient.
3. What information must be known before a drug concentration can be interpreted?
4. List some reasons why drug concentrations cannot be fully interpreted by pharmacists and doctors.
5. When might a drug concentration known to have been taken at the correct time still have been inappropriately requested?
6. If a patient's drug concentration is genuinely twice the normal maximum, in addition to reducing the dose what else should the pharmacist normally advise?

- Nunney J, Raynor DK. How are multi-compartment compliance aids used in primary care? *Pharm J* 2001; 267: 784–789. (ONLINE)
- Dodds LJ, ed. *Drugs in Use*, 3rd edn. London: Pharmaceutical Press; 2003. Chapter 32: Medicines management.

Further reading: moving on

- Green CF, McCloskey S. UK survey of the provision of multi-compartment compliance aids and medicine reminder charts on discharge from hospital. *Int J Pharm Pract* 2005; 13: 85–90. (ONLINE)
- Medicines Partnership website. *What is Concordance?* (ONLINE)

Guidance

Department of Health. *Management of Medicines – A resource to support implementation of the wider aspects of medicines management for the National Service Frameworks for Diabetes, Renal Services and Long-term Conditions* (2004). London: Department of Health; 2004.

Pharmaceutical 3 problem: the patient has difficulties with compliance

Objectives of this section

The reader should be able to detail:
- reasons for poor compliance
- strategies for improving compliance
- the difference between compliance and concordance
- the types of compliance aid available.

Further reading: basics

- Nunney J, Raynor DK. Multi-compartment compliance aids: the fact and the fiction. *Prescriber* 2003; 14: 16–21. (ONLINE)

Self-assessment questions:
Pharmaceutical 3

(Answers on p. 153)

1. What is the difference between compliance, adherence and concordance?
2. Why do patients fail to comply with their prescribed medicines?
3. What can a pharmacist do to improve compliance?
4. What are the problems with combination preparations?
5. What is a multicompartment compliance aid (MCA)?
6. What are the drawbacks to compliance aids?
7. Are there any practical alternatives to MCAs?

Chart 2.28 Pharmaceutical 3 problem: the patient has difficulties with compliance

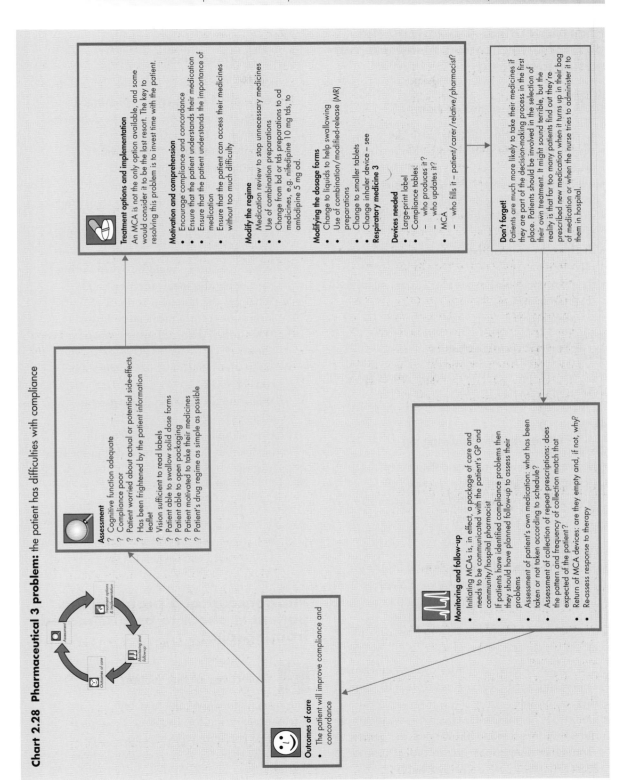

Assessment

? Cognitive function adequate
? Compliance poor
? Patient worried about actual or potential side-effects
? Has been frightened by the patient information leaflet
? Vision sufficient to read labels
? Patient able to swallow solid dose forms
? Patient able to open packaging
? Patient motivated to take their medicines
? Patient's drug regime as simple as possible

Treatment options and implementation

An MCA is not the only option available, and some would consider it to be the last resort. The key to resolving this problem is to invest time with the patient.

Motivation and comprehension

- Encourage compliance and concordance
- Ensure that the patient understands their medication
- Ensure that the patient understands the importance of medication
- Ensure that the patient can access their medicines without too much difficulty

Modify the regime

- Medication review to stop unnecessary medicines
- Use of combination preparations
- Change from bd or tds preparations to od medicines, e.g. nifedipine 10 mg tds, to amlodipine 5 mg od.

Modifying the dosage forms

- Change to liquids to help swallowing
- Use of combination/modified-release (MR) preparations
- Change to smaller tablets
- Change inhaler device – see **Respiratory medicine 3**

Devices needed

- Large-print label
- Compliance tables:
  – who produces it ?
  – who updates it?
- MCA
  – who fills it – patient/carer/relative/pharmacist?

Don't forget!

Patients are much more likely to take their medicines if they are part of the decision-making process in the first place. Patients should be involved in the selection of their own treatment. It might sound terrible, but the reality is that far too many patients find out they're prescribed new medication when it turns up in their bag of medication or when the nurse tries to administer it to them in hospital.

Monitoring and follow-up

- Initiating MCAs is, in effect, a package of care and needs to be communicated with the patient's GP and community/hospital pharmacist
- If patients have identified compliance problems then they should have planned follow-up to assess their problems
- Assessment of patient's own medication: what has been taken or not taken according to schedule?
- Assessment of collection of repeat prescriptions: does the pattern and frequency of collection match that expected of the patient?
- Return of MCA devices: are they empty and, if not, why?
- Re-assess response to therapy

Outcomes of care

- The patient will improve compliance and concordance

Pharmaceutical 4 problem: the patient's medication history is not easily identified

 Objectives of this section

The reader should be able to detail:

- the importance of good medication history taking
- why medication histories are not easily obtained from some patients, or contain errors
- the communication skills required to take histories effectively
- the sources of information available to pharmacists
- the pharmaceutical issues that can be identified by pharmacists.

 Further reading: basics

See **Problem identification and prioritisation PI3** in this book (p. 5).

 Further reading: moving on

- United Kingdom Psychiatric Pharmacy Group/University of Aston. *Expanded Medication History Form/Patient Interview.* Birmingham: United Kingdom Psychiatric Pharmacy Group/University of Aston; 2001. (ONLINE)
- Medicines Partnership. *Assessment Tool for Patients' Medicine-taking Support Needs.* London: Medicines Partnership; 2003. (ONLINE)
- Tulip SC, Cheung P, Campbell D, Walters P. Pharmaceutical care for older people: recording and review of medication following admission to hospital. *Int J Pharm Pract* 2002; 10 (Suppl): R58. (ONLINE)
- Collins D, Nickless GD, Green CF. Medication histories: does anyone know what the patient should be taking? *Int J Pharm Pract* 2004; 12: 173–178. (ONLINE – abstract only)

 Self-assessment questions: Pharmaceutical 4

(Answers on p. 155)

1. Why are pharmacists and pharmacy technicians well placed to take patients' medication histories?
2. Why is the taking of an accurate medication history important?
3. Are errors in prescribing patients' medicines on admission important, and if so why?
4. How should a patient be approached for a medication history?
5. What questions should be asked during the taking of a medication history?
6. What are the potential sources of information for a medication history?
7. What other 'medications' should be asked about?
8. What pharmaceutical issues should be considered?
9. What should be done about patients' allergies?
10. How should issues arising from the medication history be recorded in the case-notes?

Pharmaceutical 5 problem: the patient is about to be discharged from hospital

 Objectives of this section

The reader should be able to detail:

- why preparation for discharge is essential
- the most common pharmaceutical care problems that can arise at discharge from hospital

Chart 2.29 Pharmaceutical 4 problem: the patient's medication history is not easily identified

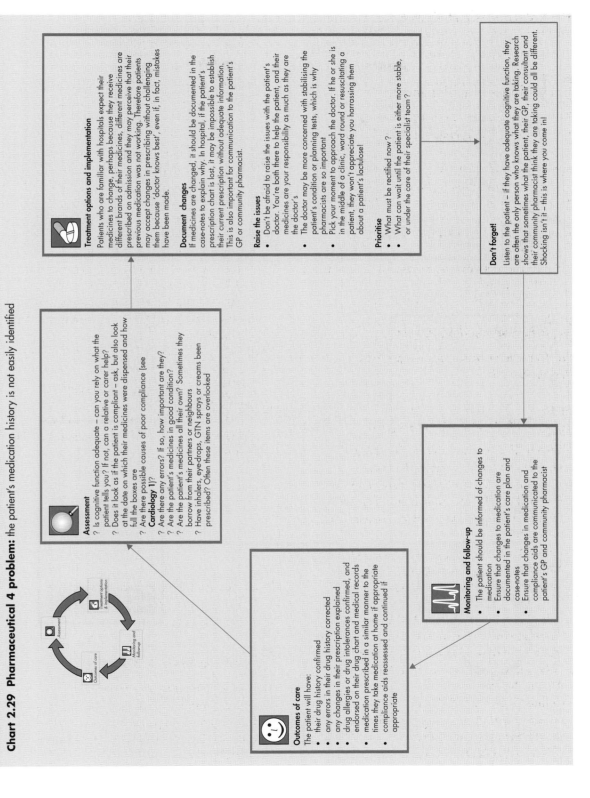

Assessment

? Is cognitive function adequate – can you rely on what the patient tells you? If not, can a relative or carer help?

? Does it look as if the patient is compliant – ask, but also look at the date on which their medicines were dispensed and how full the boxes are

? Are there possible causes of poor compliance [see **Cardiology 1**]?

? Are there any errors? If so, how important are they?

? Are the patient's medicines in good condition?

? Are the patient's medicines all their own? Sometimes they borrow from their partners or neighbours

? Have inhalers, eye-drops, GTN sprays or creams been prescribed? Often these items are overlooked

Treatment options and implementation

Patients who are familiar with hospitals expect their medicines to change, perhaps because they receive different brands of their medicines, different medicines are prescribed on admission and they may perceive that their previous medication was not working. Therefore patients may accept changes in prescribing without challenging them because 'doctor knows best', even if, in fact, mistakes have been made.

Document changes

If medicines are changed, it should be documented in the case-notes to explain why. In hospital, if the patient's prescription chart is lost, it may be impossible to establish their current prescription without adequate information. This is also important for communication to the patient's GP or community pharmacist.

Raise the issues

• Don't be afraid to raise the issues with the patient's doctor. You're both there to help the patient, and their medicines are your responsibility as much as they are the doctor's

• The doctor may be more concerned with stabilising the patient's condition or planning tests, which is why pharmacists are so important

• Pick your moment to approach the doctor. If he or she is in the middle of a clinic, ward round or resuscitating a patient, they won't appreciate you harrassing them about a patient's lactulose!

Prioritise

• What must be rectified now?

• What can wait until the patient is either more stable, or under the care of their specialist team?

Don't forget!

Listen to the patient – if they have adequate cognitive function, they are often the only person who knows what they are taking. Research shows that sometimes what the patient, their GP, their consultant and their community pharmacist think they are taking could all be different. Shocking isn't it – this is where you come in!

Monitoring and follow-up

• The patient should be informed of changes to medication

• Ensure that changes to medication are documented in the patient's care plan and case-notes

• Ensure that changes in medication and compliance aids are communicated to the patient's GP and community pharmacist

Outcomes of care

The patient will have:

• their drug history confirmed

• any errors in their drug history corrected

• any changes in their prescription explained

• drug allergies or drug intolerances confirmed, and endorsed on their drug chart and medical records

• medication prescribed in a similar manner to the times they take medication at home if appropriate

• compliance aids reassessed and continued if appropriate

Chart 2.30 Pharmaceutical 5 problem: the patient is about to be discharged from hospital

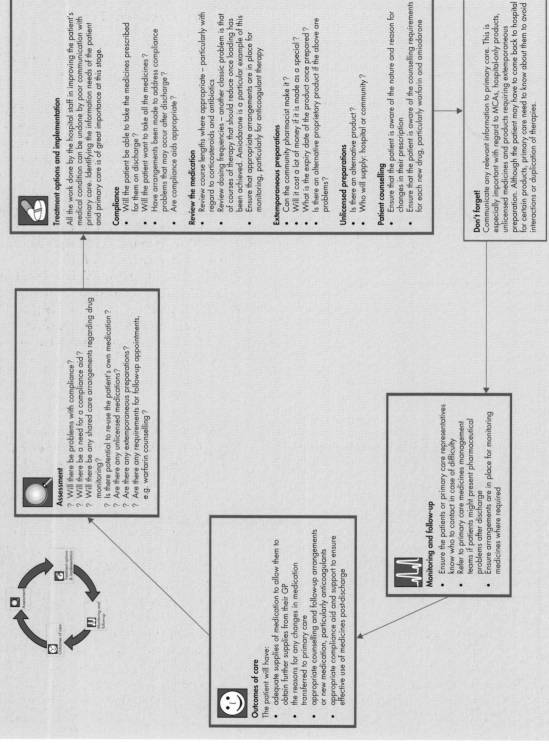

Treatment options and implementation

All the work done by the hospital staff in improving the patient's medical condition can be undone by poor communication with primary care. Identifying the information needs of the patient and primary care is of great importance at this stage.

Compliance
- Will the patient be able to take the medicines prescribed for them on discharge ?
- Will the patient want to take all the medicines ?
- Have arrangements been made to address compliance problems that may occur after discharge ?
- Are compliance aids appropriate ?

Review the medication
- Review course lengths where appropriate – particularly with regard to corticosteroids and antibiotics
- Review dosing frequencies – another classic problem is that of courses of therapy that should reduce once loading has been achieved. Amiodarone is a particular example of this
- Ensure that appropriate arrangements are in place for monitoring, particularly for anticoagulant therapy

Extemporaneous preparations
- Can the community pharmacist make it ?
- Will it cost a lot of money if it is made as a special ?
- What is the expiry date of the product once prepared ?
- Is there an alternative proprietary product if the above are problems ?

Unlicensed preparations
- Is there an alternative product ?
- Who will supply: hospital or community ?

Patient counselling
- Ensure that the patient is aware of the nature and reason for changes in their prescription
- Ensure that the patient is aware of the counselling requirements for each new drug, particularly warfarin and amiodarone

Assessment
- ? Will there be problems with compliance ?
- ? Will there be a need for a compliance aid ?
- ? Will there be any shared care arrangements regarding drug monitoring ?
- ? Is there potential to re-use the patient's own medication ?
- ? Are there any unlicensed medications ?
- ? Are there any extemporaneous preparations ?
- ? Are there any requirements for follow-up appointments, e.g. warfarin counselling ?

Don't forget!

Communicate any relevant information to primary care. This is especially important with regard to MCAs, hospital-only products, unlicensed medicines and products requiring extemporaneous preparation. Although the patient may have to come back to hospital for certain products, primary care need to know about them to avoid interactions or duplication of therapies.

Monitoring and follow-up
- Ensure the patients or primary care representatives know who to contact in case of difficulty
- Refer to primary care medicines management teams if patients might present pharmaceutical problems after discharge
- Ensure arrangements are in place for monitoring medicines where required

Outcomes of care

The patient will have:
- adequate supplies of medication to allow them to obtain further supplies from their GP
- the reasons for any changes in medication transferred to primary care
- appropriate counselling and follow-up arrangements or new medication, particularly anticoagulants
- appropriate compliance aid and support to ensure effective use of medicines post-discharge

Assessment

Treatment options
& implementation

Monitoring and
follow-up

Outcomes of care

- the patients who are in most need of pharmacists' attention
- the strategies that pharmacists can adopt to assure seamless care at hospital discharge.

 Further reading: basics

- Jackson C, Rowe P, Lea R. Pharmaceutical discharge – a professional necessity for the 1990s. *Pharm J* 1993; 250: 58–59.
- Sexton J, Ho YJ, Green CF, Caldwell NA. Ensuring seamless care at hospital discharge – a national survey. *J Clin Pharm Ther* 2000; 25: 385–393. (ONLINE – abstract only)
- Rose D, Evans SW, Williams R. Introducing a technician discharge prescription transcribing service. *Hosp Pharm* 2005; 12: 233–236. (ONLINE)

 Self-assessment questions: Pharmaceutical 5
(Answers on p.157)

1. Why is it important to communicate with primary care after discharge from hospital?
2. How should hospitals inform GPs of the changes in therapy and other important information on hospital discharge, and what problems occur in this process?
3. How much supply of medicines should a patient be given on hospital discharge?
4. Why do unlicensed medicines sometimes create problems after discharge?
5. What special attention do warfarin and other anticoagulants need after discharge?
6. Why should hospitals inform primary care about compliance aids?
7. Why do problems still occur even if hospitals inform GPs of changes in medication, unlicensed medicines and devices used?

 Answers to self-assessment questions: Pharmaceutical 1: adverse drug reactions (p. 137)

1. **What is the definition of an ADR?**
The World Health Organization definition of an ADR is: 'A response to a drug which is noxious and unintended and which occurs at doses normally used in man for the prophylaxis, diagnosis or therapy of disease or for the modification of a physiological function' (see 'Further reading: moving on' for **P1**). Note that this definition excludes intentional or non-intentional overdose or poisoning.

2. **Why are ADRs a problem?**
ADRs are a problem because they cause hospital admissions, delay cure of the disease that they were intended to treat, complicate existing disease, may result in inappropriate treatment or investigations, affect quality of life and increase health costs. Coverage of ADRs, for example, with regard to the COX-2 inhibitors can cause patients to lose confidence in medicines. Adverse publicity over the measles, mumps and rubella (MMR) vaccine has led to a decrease in uptake of the vaccine, which may result in an increase in the diseases that they were designed to prevent.

3. **What is the incidence of ADRs?**
The incidence of ADRs depends on where you look and on the nature of the patients, for example, young or old, surgical or medical. In community settings there are

(Continued)

no data, but in hospitals it is thought that 10–20% of inpatients suffer ADRs, 6.7% suffer 'serious' ADRs, 5% of admissions are ADR related and 0.25–3% of deaths are due to ADRs.

4. **Should drugs that aren't safe be prevented from being marketed?**

Ideally yes, but clinical trials have limitations in that they are small in size, select particular groups of patients with specific illnesses and exclude others on a similar basis. They may restrict concurrent drug therapy and be short in duration. This means that once a drug is launched onto the open market it is exposed to a number of new situations that may result in an adverse drug reaction, interaction or drug–disease interaction.

5. **What is the difference between type A and type B reactions?**

Type A reactions tend to augment effects of the drug's known pharmacology. They are usually predictable, usually dose related and have a high morbidity but a low mortality. Type B reactions tend to be bizarre, unpredictable, unrelated to dose, with low morbidity but high mortality. This is important to understand because, in the case of type A reactions, a reduction in dose may well result in resolution of the ADR, but, in the case of type B reactions, the drug should be withdrawn.

6. **Which groups of drugs are most commonly associated with ADRs?**

All drugs have some risk of ADRs, but of particular importance are those that have a narrow therapeutic index, most commonly digoxin, theophylline, gentamicin and lithium, and particularly in combination with non-linear kinetics, for example phenytoin. Also, any medicines with potential for interaction should be closely monitored, for example warfarin, antiepileptics and quinolone antibiotics.

A number of drug classes are known to have clinically important adverse effects and these should be closely monitored, for example antirheumatic drugs, immunosuppressants, antithyroid drugs, cytotoxics, NSAIDs, diuretics and corticosteroids.

7. **Why are elderly people at increased risk of experiencing an ADR?**

Some elderly patients are unfortunate enough to experience multiple pathologies, and as a result may be required to take more and more medicines and thus suffer from polypharmacy. As a result, the likelihood of an ADR, drug–drug or drug–disease interaction increases too. Furthermore, ageing results in important pharmacokinetic and pharmacodynamic changes which result in altered drug metabolism and excretion, altered organ sensitivity and decreased functional and homeostatic reserve, that is, the effects of medication may be more pronounced in an elderly patient.

8. **Why is it difficult to detect ADRs?**

Often, the first problem is that an ADR is never even considered as a cause of the patient's problems. Beyond that, the ADR may not be associated with current medication, ADRs may masquerade as other diseases and there are few clinical or laboratory methods of testing for them. Biopsies, therapeutic drug monitoring and laboratory data may provide important clues, but there are few definitive tests available.

9. **What are the purposes of post-marketing surveillance?**

The main purposes of post-marketing surveillance are to detect previously unrecognised ADRs, identify risk factors for ADRs in individual patients, collate data concerning recognised ADRs and

$\rightarrow$

compare the safety of drugs within the same class.

10. **For what reasons do healthcare professionals often fail to report ADRs?**
Lack of awareness of the existence of an ADR is the first problem. Other issues include familiarity with a drug or common adverse effect, lack of confidence that an ADR has occurred, concern about confidentiality for the patient, or lack of time, lethargy and complacency or, sometimes, professionals feel guilty because of patient suffering. With less than 10% of serious ADRs being reported, there is a massive amount of drug safety data that goes unrecognised, which could be used to improve the safe use of medicines.

11. **What can the MHRA do about ADRs?**
The MHRA can write to healthcare professionals on an individual basis to warn them of specific problems. *Current Problems* is a bulletin used to highlight drug safety issues, and the MHRA can also publish reports in letters, journals and press releases. With regard to the medicines themselves, the MHRA can insist on amendments to summaries of product characteristics, insist on withdrawal of medicines from the market, and publish highlighted warnings in the *BNF*, for example for NSAIDs or antithyroid agents.

12. **What are the limitations of CSM data?**
Because of gross under-reporting, only a fraction of the data is available to work with, and thus it is impossible to calculate incidence rates. ADRs, which are well publicised, often become more frequently reported, as may ADRs that occur in medicines that are reported to be safer, for example, GI bleeds with COX-2 inhibitors. As a result, CSM data can be used only to generate hypotheses about drug safety that require further investigation where appropriate.

13. **What are the responsibilities of the pharmacist with regard to ADRs?**
First, the pharmacist needs to be proactive in monitoring patients for ADRs, and should ensure that other healthcare professionals are aware of this. Monitoring is vital, particularly of risk drugs, risk patients and black triangle drugs, which are newly launched medicines for which the CSM requires all ADRs to be reported, whether serious or not. Pharmacists also need to ensure that they are aware of the adverse effects of all the medicines that their patients are taking. Finally, it is an important role of the pharmacist to report the adverse effects of drugs using the MHRA/CSM Yellow Card scheme.

**Answers to self-assessment questions:
Pharmaceutical 2: narrow
therapeutic index drugs** (p. 144)

1. **Do all drugs for which plasma concentrations can be obtained require concentrations to be measured?**
No, only for those drugs:
   • with a narrow therapeutic range such as gentamicin, theophylline, etc., where the

drug concentration likely to produce the desired clinical effect is very close to the concentration that may cause side-effects and harm
   • for which there is a clear relationship between concentration and clinical effect
   • where there is suspected toxicity or subtherapeutic response, or poor adherence to the prescribed regime.

(Continued)

2. **Give some justifiable reasons for requesting a drug concentration measurement to be obtained from a patient.**

Before the decision to measure serum drug concentrations can be supported, the question should be asked, 'Will the result change the clinical management of the patient?'. If it will not, then it could be that there is no justifiable reason for requesting the blood concentration to be measured. Concentrations are requested for a variety of reasons, from 'Why not?' to much more valid reasons; to check compliance, investigate the possibility of dose-related side-effects; to examine the potential effects of a pharmacokinetic drug interaction, test the validity of a loading dose and many others. There are also situations where the taking of concentrations is an essential part of care, for example measuring ciclosporin levels after renal transplantation.

3. **What information must be known before a drug concentration can be interpreted?**

The meaningful interpretation of a drug concentration requires some relevant information:

- the clinical indication of the prescribed drug
- the recent and relevant dosage history: what was administered and when. This would include what happened over the last five half-lives, whereas what happened a year ago would clearly be irrelevant in most situations
- the route of administration and dosage form used
- the sample time in relation to the administration time of the drug.

It might be harmful to the patient to adjust their dose based on incomplete information. For example, if a patient had a low serum concentration of a drug but had recently experienced diarrhoea and vomiting affecting absorption, or had missed doses, an increase in dose would be inappropriate.

4. **List some reasons why drug concentrations cannot be fully interpreted by pharmacists and doctors.**

A common reason is that the concentration has been measured before steady state has been reached, traditionally at five half-lives after initiation or dose change, and hence interpretation is not straightforward. This could be more than a week in the case of drugs such as digoxin or phenytoin. The concentration must be taken at the appropriate time, so that ciclosporin interpretation, for example, is based on a 12-hour trough (immediately before a dose) or a 2-hour post-dose peak. Samples taken other than at these times will give distorted results, as will 'trough levels' taken after the patient has had their dose, rather than just before it.

Finally, information may not have been recorded by the person who took the sample. A typical scenario in hospital is reviewing a reported gentamicin concentration of 4 mg/L. With no other information this could be a high trough, a low peak or simply a random concentration. Patients in these situations can be an invaluable source of the missing information, especially if briefed beforehand to note down the times of drug administration and sampling.

5. **When might a drug concentration known to have been taken at the correct time still have been inappropriately requested?**

If, whatever the result obtained by the laboratory, no doctor will be willing to change a drug dose, then the inconvenience to the patient and costs to the laboratory will have been in vain. Examples of this include requesting theophylline concentrations in patients on doses that will be expected to be subtherapeutic, in

$\longrightarrow$

hospitals where it is not convention to aim for the standard target ranges, or where patients are displaying no signs of toxicity or suboptimal response. Alternatively, for drugs such as digoxin, if the symptoms are controlled, the dose looks appropriate for the patient's renal function and there are no signs of toxicity, then monitoring drug concentrations is probably unnecessary. However, if toxicity were suspected, concentrations should be measured.

6. **If a patient's drug concentration is genuinely twice the normal maximum, in addition to reducing the dose what else should the pharmacist normally advise?**
Unless there are particular clinical circumstances that make it inappropriate, most pharmacists would advise omitting doses in these circumstances.

Answers to self-assessment questions: Pharmaceutical 3: difficulties with compliance (p. 144)

1. **What is the difference between compliance, adherence and concordance?**
Compliance was originally used as a blunt measure of how a patient performed in terms of taking their medication. This was a basic comparison of the number of tablets actually taken with the number that the patient might have been expected to take. Like the similar term 'adherence', it has expanded to include when and how medication is taken. Compliance is very difficult to measure, and often, by adopting a non-judgemental approach, pharmacists can encourage honesty on the part of patients. Concordance does not express compliance, but is described on the Medicines Partnership website as a 'process of prescribing and medicine taking based on partnership'. A patient can therefore not be non-concordant, but the relationship between them and their carers can be. Thus if a patient's blood pressure therapy makes them dizzy and leads to non-compliance, because the doctor has insisted that the patient continue with therapy regardless, then the doctor–patient relationship is 'non-concordant.'

2. **Why do patients fail to comply with their prescribed medication regime?**
This can be inadvertent – if the regime is complicated, the patient is muddled or forgetful, or there is simply poor understanding about why, when and how medicines are to be taken. Alternatively, it may be the result of a decision by the patient in response to perceptions about their condition, the medication or their carers. Therapy may have caused adverse events, or have produced no tangible benefits, or the leaflet in the pack may have frightened them. Education and the promotion of concordance may overcome some of these decisions.

3. **What can a pharmacist do to improve compliance?**
Recognition of the above leads to the identification of roles for pharmacists in helping patients manage their medicines. Steps that can be taken to improve compliance include:

(Continued)

- assess cognitive ability to comply with dosing instructions
- rationalise dosing regime – use modified-release or combination dosage forms
- counsel regarding adverse effects and what to expect from medicines
- change to liquids or smaller tablets if swallowing is a problem
- use large print labels for those with visual impairment
- use compliance charts or multicompartment compliance aids
- supply aids that assist eye-drop and inhaler use, or the removal of tablets from containers.

4. **What are the problems with combination preparations?**

There are a few problems with combination preparations. The combination may not be logical. For example, co-proxamol contained a quantity of paracetamol that resulted in patients not receiving the maximum dose of paracetamol in 24 hours, in fact one-third less. Combinations may also be more expensive and are often used as a ploy by some manufacturers to extend their products' patent length or marketing lifetime. Combinations may result in less flexibility around dosing if the individual components need to be adjusted separately, for example with inhaler therapy.

5. **What is a multicompartment compliance aid (MCA)?**

In the UK the available MCA devices vary in size and structure; some are disposable, whereas others are reusable. Most have a division of the aid into seven days of the week, and each day into four or more sections representing dosing times. Reusable MCAs, for example the 'Dosett' box, tend to be constructed of plastic with sliding covers to facilitate both the dispensing and extraction of medicines. Disposable MCAs, for example the 'Venalink' system, usually consist of a card sheet, with plastic blisters backed with foil, which can be broken by the patient in a similar fashion to a standard blister pack found in original manufacturers' packaging.

6. **What are the drawbacks to compliance aids?**

Surprisingly, there is little evidence that MCAs improve compliance in most patients. In comparison to standard (and particularly original pack) dispensing, the provision of medicines in MCAs can be time-consuming. Because of the size of the MCAs and the volume of medicines placed in them, it can be difficult to detect dispensing errors. Other areas of concern include the stability of medicines that, once removed from their original packaging, may become unstable and cannot be dispensed in an MCA. Furthermore, some MCAs may be difficult to open or manipulate for patients with manual dexterity problems, and it has been argued that MCAs may reduce opportunities for patients to learn about their medicines, because they are simply following the MCA instructions.

7. **Are there any practical alternatives to MCAs?**

Alternatives to MCAs such as tailoring dosing times to fit with patients' routines, and using medicines reminder charts (MRCs) may be of benefit. The MRCs used in the UK generally include a list of the patient's medicines with columns for times of day when the doses are to be taken. Some also include the purpose of the medicine. Other methods of improving compliance include telephone reminders, timed alarms, tick box labels and refrigerator stickers.

Answers to self-assessment questions:
**Pharmaceutical 4: drug history
problems** (p. 146)

1. **Why are pharmacists and pharmacy
technicians well placed to take patients'
medication histories?**
Pharmacists and pharmacy technicians have
the best understanding of medicines and
their formulations. They are therefore in a
good position to assess potential problems
related to medicines, and identify potential
or actual medicines-related problems
causing admission.

2. **Why is the taking of an accurate medication
history important?**
Errors occur when medication histories are
taken on admission to hospital. This is for a
variety of reasons, but mostly because the
number of areas that a doctor is expected to
evaluate means that, depending on
experience, the condition of the patient and
distractions around them, it may be difficult
for the doctor to evaluate the patient's
medication history. As a result of these
errors, medications are therefore missing,
added in or incorrectly prescribed in terms
of dose, formulation or dosing schedule.

3. **Are errors in prescribing patients' medicines
on admission important, and if so why?**
Yes, these errors are important. Prescribing
errors may influence the effect of drug
interactions, confuse the patient, include
cautions or contraindications, or result in
adverse drug reactions. Errors are also a
problem because they may not be noticed;
patients accept changes as normal for
hospital and they may result in
inappropriate treatment or management, or
an extended stay in hospital.

4. **How should a patient be approached for a
medication history?**

The first thing that should be done is to
introduce yourself, say your name, what
you do and why you are going to speak to
the patient. Your visit may not be expected,
so reassure the patient that you're not going
to examine them, but talk about their
medicines. Create a comfortable
environment – be friendly and relaxed but
remain professional. Avoid the use of jargon
– it can confuse the patient. One of the
most important things is to listen – be
receptive to the patient. Never dismiss
things that they say out of hand – you may
be missing vital information.

5. **What questions should be asked during the
taking of a medication history?**
There is no set list of questions but points
that should be covered include:
- are you taking any medicines prescribed
by your GP?
- have you got them with you?
- who looks after your medicines (often it
may be a partner or son or daughter)
- is there anything that you'd like to ask
about your medicines?
- do you have any problems with your
medicines?
- do you experience any side-effects from
your medicines?
Sample data-collection forms can be found
in the ONLINE links.

6. **What are the potential sources of
information for a medication history?**
The patient or their relative or carer should
be the primary source. Additional
information can be obtained from their
repeat prescription if they have one. GPs
may provide an admission letter and,
increasingly, these letters contain a list of
recently prescribed medicines, but these
should be interpreted cautiously since they

(Continued)

may contain medicines prescribed as a one-off, or discontinued. These lists often are copied directly onto a medication chart and so should be checked carefully. Nursing home medication administration records (MAR sheets) are also a good source of information and usually include whether a patient has actually been administered, although not necessarily taken, their medication. Community pharmacists are also a good source, but it should be borne in mind that not every patient uses the same one. Finally, previous admission records are a potential source of information, but, again, may be incorrect if the GP or clinic has made changes to the patient's medication.

7. **What other 'medications' should be asked about?**

OTC medicine purchases should be investigated as should herbal or Chinese medication. Smoking tobacco, drinking alcohol and illicit drug use should also be explored as they may have significant impacts on conventional drug therapy or cardiovascular risk. Finally, again, be sure to question the use of oral contraceptive 'pills' since patients may not view these as important, even though they are. The same applies to eye-drops, injections and inhalers.

8. **What pharmaceutical issues should be considered?**

Dosage form can be important; inhalers and sprays and similar devices are often wrongly prescribed. Modified-release preparations and enteric-coated (EC) preparations are often incorrectly prescribed too.

9. **What should be done about patients' allergies?**

The patient should be asked about any drug allergies, and where they are identified the nature of the allergy should be explored. Patients often confuse drug intolerance with true allergy, and in these situations intolerance labelled as allergy may deny a patient potentially life-saving therapy. Any findings from these questions should be clearly documented in the patient's case-notes and medication chart.

10. **How should issues arising from the medication history be recorded in the case-notes?**

Most organisations have their own guidelines but most standards recommend that entries should:

- state the date and time of the entry
- insert a heading making the purpose of entry visible, in this case 'Pharmacist re: Medication history' might be appropriate
- state the nature of the entry, that is, say what has been done and make a clear note of the problem
- make the required action clear – the reader needs to understand, in clear language, what needs to be done
- sign and print your name and insert some contact details, usually a pager or telephone number.

Under no circumstances must you put in writing any comments that are critical of practice, be judgmental or sensationalist, or direct the action of a clinician. Case-notes may be used as a source of evidence in an inquest or court proceeding and you must make sure that you do not enter anything in case-notes or behave in a manner that could be open to criticism.

Answers to self-assessment questions:
Pharmaceutical 5: discharge from
hospital (p. 149)

1. **Why is it important to communicate with primary care after discharge from hospital?**
This is important because any changes made to a patient's medication need to be transferred to their primary care record. If this were not to happen, it would be quite likely that the patient would end up taking the medicines that they were previously prescribed, prior to their hospital admission. Also, there may be prescribing quality issues around dosing or drug selection that contributed to the patient's admission, which should be communicated to the patient's GP.

2. **How should hospitals inform GPs of the changes in therapy and other important information on hospital discharge, and what problems occur in this process?**
Most hospitals have a combined discharge prescription and discharge note for the GP. Much work over the last 20 years shows that no one method of communication is perfect. If the patient has a copy of this note, this may be the most effective method of communication, but only if the patient passes it to the GP. In addition it might cause worries if the patient reads sensitive information on it.

   Alternatively, the hospital can post, fax or courier a copy to the GP. But whose job is this? In many hospitals this falls to ward clerks, but delays in the system mean that the patient may present to their doctor for follow-up before this has happened. Some hospitals have passed this role to the pharmacy department but it can work only if the junior doctor has remembered to fill in the GP details, and hospital managers are happy to transfer resources into the pharmacy department to fund the labour required. A few hospitals use both

approaches together – a copy to be patient carried and another to be sent direct to the doctor in primary care in a 'belt-and-braces' approach.

3. **How much supply of medicines should a patient be given on hospital discharge?**
Traditionally, only a 7-day supply of medication was given in most UK hospitals, which involved both a lot of cutting of foil strips in the dispensary, and patients running out of therapy before their GP could see them. With the rise of original pack dispensing, many hospitals now give up to 28 days' supply of medication, but this does require a transfer of resources into the hospitals from the primary care purchasers. Of course, if a patient is on antibiotics or steroids, for example, shorter courses may well be appropriate.

4. **Why do unlicensed medicines sometimes create problems after discharge?**
Unlicensed medicines are a problem in that they tend to require some specialist knowledge of the drug concerned, use of the drug and how to obtain them from wholesalers. For these reasons, GPs may be unwilling to prescribe them and community pharmacists may be unwilling to attempt to obtain them.

5. **What special attention do warfarin and other anticoagulants need after discharge?**
Warfarin has a narrow therapeutic index, and interacts with a number of other drugs and foodstuffs. For this reason, patients need careful counselling about the potential for interaction, how to take doses, and what the signs of excessive anticoagulation might be. Adequate arrangements need to be in place to ensure that the patient is monitored appropriately and has access to support if necessary.

6. **Why should hospitals inform primary care about compliance aids?**

(Continued)

Where compliance aids are in use, primary care practitioners need to be aware of their existence in case of a change in medication that will require adjustment to the contents or labelling of a device or table respectively. It will also highlight the need for the patient to have support with their medicines-taking practices. In some cases, arrangements will be required for the patient to have their compliance aid filled by the community pharmacist, and

again this requires prior agreement and planning.

7. **Why do problems still occur even if hospitals inform GPs of changes in medication, unlicensed medicines and devices used?**

It may be that a busy surgery simply fails to act proactively on all the information communicated to them. However, in the absence of patient registration with particular pharmacies, hospitals often have great difficulty, even if they were willing and able to, in informing community pharmacies of the information that they would need to ensure seamless care.

Section 3

Examples of Pharmaceutical Care Planning

Introduction

Case study examples

The following cases aim to illustrate how to construct a pharmaceutical care plan for a patient with multiple problems, by using the model described in Section 1 and the pathways described in Section 2. It should be remembered that the individual drug choices made in the model answers are not necessarily the only possible answers – different NHS trusts/PCTs may have a different first-line agent within the same class, or patients may require different choices in the light of their history and co-morbidities.

Terminology

In the cases, the standard UK abbreviations are used to describe the case:

- **PC: presenting complaint** – the reason why the patient has presented to their doctor or hospital, or been sent for pharmaceutical care review. It can be both narrow, e.g. the patient is fitting, or broad, e.g. where the patient has an exacerbation of COPD
- **HPC: history of the presenting complaint** – the events that led up to the presenting complaint, which may take two lines or several pages to describe
- **PMH: previous medical history** – other relevant history, co-morbidity and so forth, as completely recorded as possible. In hospital admissions, the admitting doctor may be able to glean only the briefest of details at the time that they are 'clerking-in' the patient
- **DHx: medication (drug) history** – usually this is little more than a list of the currently taken medication and allergies. Much work shows how frequently this is incorrect in the records of both primary and secondary care physicians, and is rarely trusted completely by pharmacists
- **FHx/SHx: family history/social history** – relevant history, reasons for death of parents/close family members, care environment for vulnerable patients, smoking and alcohol habits etc.

- **ROS/O/E: review of systems/on examination** – the practitioner will first briefly enquire, in a logical sequence, about the patient's various body systems, and then examine the patient in the same order
- **impression/plan** – the above lead into the doctor, pharmacist or nurse deciding to do further tests or come to a diagnosis or, more likely, an impression of the patient's problems.

Case 1: a patient who has presented to their local accident and emergency department with haematemesis

- **Patient:** Mr TR, 57 years old
- **PC:** haematemesis (vomiting blood)
- **HPC:** been vomiting for past 2 days. Today noticed coffee-ground appearance with some fresh blood. No melaena (blood in stools)
- **PMH:**
  — rheumatoid arthritis
  — congestive heart failure
  — hypertension
- **DHx:**
  — methotrexate 15 mg weekly
  — folic acid 5 mg once weekly
  — naproxen 500 mg bd
  — lisinopril 20 mg od
  — frusemide 40 mg od
  — no known drug allergies (NKDA)
- **O/E:**
  — BP = 105/68 mmHg, pulse = 98 beats/minute
  — abdomen soft, non-tender
- **Impression:** upper GI bleed
- **Initial blood tests** (normal range in parentheses):
  — urea = 8.8 mmol/L (<7.5)
  — creatinine (Cr) = 110 micromoles/L (<110)
  — haemoglobin (Hb) = 9.7 g/dL (13.5–16.5)
  — mean cell volume (MCV) = 76 fL (80–96)
  — remainder: NAD (nothing adverse detected)
- **Plan:**
  — OGD (which shows a superficial duodenal ulcer)
  — start PPI.

Initial assessment: pharmaceutical care problems identified

- Haematemesis due to duodenal ulcer
- Rheumatoid arthritis
- Congestive heart failure
- Hypertension
- Anaemia.

Problem prioritisation for action by the pharmacist

1. Duodenal ulcer with haematemesis: reason for admission
2. Anaemia: due to bleeding ulcer?
3. Rheumatoid arthritis: currently controlled?
4. Congestive heart failure: well controlled?
5. Hypertension: currently well below targets.

Case 2: a patient who has presented with chest pains

- **Patient:** Mrs CB, 48 years old
- **PC:** chest pain
- **HPC:**
  - retrosternal chest pain, tight in nature
  - worse on exertion
- **PMH:**
  - type 2 DM
  - hypertension
  - angina
  - asthma (only uses salbutamol occasionally)
- **DHx:**
  - metformin 850 mg tds
  - gliclazide 80 mg bd
  - bendroflumethiazide 2.5 mg od
  - salbutamol 2 puffs prn
  - beclometasone 200 micrograms, 2 puffs bd
  - GTN spray 1–2 puffs prn
- **SHx:** smokes 15 cigarettes per day
- **O/E:**
  - BP = 150/90 mmHg, pulse = 102/minute
  - patient obese
- **Blood tests:**
  - total cholesterol:high-density liopprotein (HDL) = 7.5
  - HbA_{1c} = 8%
  - random blood glucose = 13.3 mmol/L
- **Impression:** worsening angina, no signs of MI on ECG
- **Plan:** admit and manage.

Initial assessment: pharmaceutical care problems identified

- Chest pains (angina): symptom of ischaemic heart disease (IHD)
- Type 2 DM
- Hypertension
- Asthma
- CVD risks.

Problem prioritisation for action by pharmacist

1. IHD: highest priority as aims of treatment are not being met
2. Hypertension: high priority since aims of treatment are not being met
3. Type 2 DM: high priority since aims of treatment are not being met
4. CVD risks: hypercholesterolaemia – high priority since aims of treatment are not being met, with smoking cigarettes
5. Asthma: low priority since appears well controlled.

Case 3: a patient with a history of falls and confusion

- **Patient:** Mr AB, 77-year-old male
- **PC:** falls and increased confusion over the past few days.
- **HPC:**
  - poor historian – history from family – 'legs are giving way'
  - also complaining of quiescent headaches over the past week and occasional dizziness
  - no loss of consciousness/eye pain/visual disturbances
- **PMH:**
  - CVA 3 years ago: left hemiparesis
  - depression

Table 3.1 Pharmaceutical care plan for Mr TR

Problem	Desired outcomes of treatment ☺	Detailed assessment 🔍	Action	Follow-up and monitoring 〰
Duodenal ulcer	• Heal ulcer • Prevent relapse	• Due to naproxen? • *H. pylori* status?	• Stop naproxen • Oral PPI for 4 weeks • Eradication therapy if *H. pylori* positive	• Presence of symptoms • Rescope to confirm healing
Anaemia	• Correct Hb (target)	• Due to blood loss from ulcer? • Due to RA?	• If iron deficient, start ferrous sulphate 200 mg tds • Add ascorbic acid since also on PPI	• Hb after 2–3 months • Symptoms of anaemia (e.g. fatigue, shortness of breath)
Rheumatoid arthritis	• Prevent relapses • Control symptoms • Slow progression of disease	• Appears controlled at present • Can patient cope without NSAID?	• If patient cannot cope without NSAID, restart once ulcer healed but add in long-term PPI	• Symptom control • CRP, ESR • Functioning of joints • FBC and LFTs since on methotrexate (risk of toxicity as was on NSAID)
Congestive heart failure	• Reduce symptoms (shortness of breath, ankle swelling) • Reduce hospital admissions • Prevent premature mortality	• Symptoms appear well controlled at present • Is patient's condition stable? If so could you consider adding a beta-blocker? • Number of hospital admissions in last year? • Could lisinopril dose be titrated further?	• If stable, consider starting bisoprolol 1.25 mg initially and titrate slowly • Consider increasing dose of lisinopril if BP will allow this	• Signs of worsening oedema (e.g. ankle swelling, shortness of breath) • Pulse, BP • U+Es • Weight
Hypertension	• Control BP, target <130/80 mmHg	• BP appears controlled, but is level lower than normal due to bleed? • Lisinopril a good choice since patient also has heart failure	• Continue to monitor BP • No action required	• Monitor BP • Monitor urea, Cr, K⁺

Table 3.2 Pharmaceutical care plan for Mrs CB

Problem	Desired outcomes of treatment	Detailed assessment	Action	Follow-up and monitoring
Ischaemic heart disease	• Prevent symptoms (angina) • Prevent ACS	• Currently using GTN too often • Not receiving any prophylactic therapy	• Start aspirin 75 mg od • Start diltiazem SR 60 mg bd (beta-blocker contraindicated since asthmatic) NB: stick to same brand of diltiazem • Stop smoking	• Frequency of chest pain/GTN use • Monitor pulse and BP as diltiazem started
Type 2 DM	• Keep peripheral blood glucose (BM) 4–7 mmol/L • HbA$_{1c}$ <7% • Prevent long-term complications	• HbA$_{1c}$ not meeting target • BM too high • Patient developed one complication (angina) • BP also high • Body mass index (BMI) = obese	• Dietary advice to help lose weight • Check compliance with medicines • If compliance OK, consider increasing gliclazide dose to 120 mg bd • May need to consider insulin	• BMs qds until in range, then four times/week • HbA$_{1c}$ every 3 months • BP every 3 months
Hypertension	• Aim for BP <130/80 mmHg	• Currently a little high • Need to recheck when chest pain has settled	• Introduction of diltiazem may result in adequate control • May need to increase diltiazem dose if still not meeting target BP	• BP and pulse
CVD risk: cholesterol	• Lower cholesterol to <4 mmol/L	• Not receiving therapy currently • Since cholesterol is raised and patient diabetic, needs statin therapy	• Start simvastatin 40 mg od – counsel re: signs of rhabdomyolysis • Low-fat diet	• Recheck cholesterol in 3 months • Monitor LFTs • Patient observing for signs of rhabdomyolysis
CVD risk: smoking	• Patient to give up smoking	• Has contributed to development of angina and increases overall CVD risk • Potential to worsen asthma	• Consider nicotine replacement therapy (NRT) (can use even though cautioned in CVD as patient has not had MI) • Consider counselling	• Has patient stopped smoking?
Asthma	• Control symptoms • Reduce exacerbations	• Currently well controlled	• Check inhaler technique (always worth doing) • Consider stepping down treatment (e.g. reducing inhaled steroid dose)	• Daily peak flows • Symptom diary

Table 3.3 Pharmaceutical care plan for Mr AB

Problem	Desired outcomes of treatment	Detailed assessment	Action	Follow-up and monitoring
Falls – over past few days, confusion	• Prevent further falls • Resolve acute confusion • Prevent further confusion	• Due to nitrazepam hangover effect? • Due to SSRI-induced postural hypotension? • Due to codeine in Tylex? • Due to co-amilofruse? • Due to poor mobility as result of obesity? • Mechanical? Infection? Other?	• Convert nitrazepam to diazepam and withdraw very slowly (counsel patient and wife) • Measure lying and standing BP to see if a postural drop exists • Try non-drug measures for insomnia • Try paracetamol for pain	• Monitor for signs of withdrawal
Raised cholesterol	• Aim for cholesterol <4 mmol/L	• Not currently prescribed any treatment	• Start simvastatin 40 mg nocte • Counsel re signs of rhabdomyolysis	• Monitor cholesterol • Monitor LFTs • Patient observes for signs of rhabdomyolysis
Unnecessary medication	• Ensure all medications prescribed have a valid indication	• No valid indication for co-amilofruse?	• Stop co-amilofruse	• Monitor for signs of fluid retention
Previous CVA	• Prevent further events	• Risks: raised cholesterol, age	• Continue aspirin dose to 75 mg od • Start simvastatin 40 mg nocte	• Sign of further CVA • Cholesterol after 3 months • LFTs as statin commenced
Depression	• Improve patient's mood and wellbeing	• Post CVA?	• Continue	• Symptoms and mood
Insomnia	• Ensure patient sleeps properly	• Is fluoxetine effective? • Has he been taking fluoxetine at night? • Is pain keeping the patient awake? • Is depression affecting sleep?	• Ensure fluoxetine taken in the morning • Try non-pharmacological methods, e.g. avoid caffeine before bedtime, relaxation etc.	• Sleep diary
Pain	• Ensure adequate control of pain	• What is the cause of his pain? • Tylex causing drowsiness/confusion?	• Try regular paracetamol initially • If opiates required, start at low dose	• Pain scores
Compliance issues	• Patient will receive correct therapy once discharged	• Who manages medicines administration now? • Who obtains further supplies?	• MRC? • MCA? • Involve carers? Primary care?	• Patient feedback prior to discharge • Liaison with primary care staff

- DHx:
  — aspirin 75 mg od
  — co-amilofruse 5/40 2 tabs mane
  — nitrazepam 5–10 mg nocte
  — fluoxetine 20 mg mane
  — Tylex prn
- SHx:
  — lives with wife
  — no alcohol or smoking
- O/E:
  — alert, slightly confused, resting tremor.
  — GCS = 14/15
  — BP = 141/88 mmHg, pulse = 84 beats/minute, apyrexial
  — abdomen soft, non-tender
  — neurological examination: cranial nerves intact, left hypertonus
  — review of systems (ROS): NAD
- **Initial blood tests**: cholesterol = 6.6 mmol/L
- **Impression**: general deterioration/infection.

Initial assessment: pharmaceutical care problems identified

- Falls and confusion
- Previous CVA
- Depression
- Raised serum cholesterol
- Medication without clear indication?
- Insomnia?
- Pain?
- Compliance issues.

Problem prioritisation for action by pharmacist

1. Falls and confusion: highest priority since they are the reason for admission
2. Raised cholesterol: high priority since aims of treatment are not being met
3. Medication without indication: medium priority
4. Previous CVA: low priority
5. Depression: low priority
6. Insomnia: low priority
7. Pain: low priority.

Abbreviations

ABCD	'ACEI/ARB, beta-blocker, CCB, diuretic' (device for selecting antihypertensive in BHS 2004 Guidelines)
ACEI	angiotensin-converting enzyme inhibitor, e.g. ramipril
ACS	acute coronary syndrome
ADR	adverse drug reaction
AIDS	acquired immune deficiency syndrome
Al^{3+}	aluminium
ALT	alanine transaminase (a liver enzyme)
ALP	alkaline phosphatase (a liver enzyme)
APTT	activated partial thromboplastin time (monitors unfractionated heparin therapy)
ARB	angiotensin II receptor blocker, e.g. losartan
5-ASA	5-aminosalicylic acid
bd	twice a day
BHS	British Hypertension Society
BM	peripheral blood glucose (measured with a 'BM' stick)
BMD	bone mineral density
BMI	body mass index
BNF	*British National Formulary*
BP	blood pressure
BRAS	bilateral renal artery stenosis (contraindication to ACEIs)
BTS	British Thoracic Society
Ca^{2+}	calcium
CCB	calcium-channel blocker (see DHP-CCB/RLCCB)

CCF	congestive cardiac failure
CD	Crohn's disease
CHD	coronary heart disease
CNS	central nervous system
COPD	chronic obstructive pulmonary disease
COX	cyclo-oxygenase – enzyme with two forms
Cr	creatinine
CrCl	creatinine clearance
CRP	C-reactive protein (marker of inflammation and infection)
CSM	Committee on the Safety of Medicines
CVA	cerebrovascular accident
CVD	cardiovascular disease (coronary heart disease + cerebrovascular disease)
DAS	Disease Activity Score
DCCT	Diabetes Control and Complications Trial (for type 1 DM)
DH or DHx	medication (drug) history
DHP-CCB	dihydropyridine calcium-channel blocker, e.g. amlodipine
DMARD	disease-modifying antirheumatic drug, e.g. sulfasalazine, methotrexate
DM	diabetes mellitus – two types
DVLA	Driver and Vehicle Licensing Agency (UK)
DVT	deep vein thrombosis
EBM	evidence-based medicine
EC	enteric coated
ECG	electrocardiogram

ESR	erythrocyte sedimentation rate – marker of inflammation	MAOI	monoamine oxidase inhibitor, e.g. phenelzine
ESRF/ESRD	end-stage renal failure/disease	MAR	medication administration record
FBC	full blood count	MCA	multicompartment compliance aid
FEV_1	forced expiratory volume in 1 second	MCV	mean cell volume
		MDI	metered dose inhaler
FH or FHx	family history	MHRA	Medicines and Healthcare Products Regulatory Agency (UK)
FP10	standard prescription in England and Wales for dispensing by community pharmacists. Usually from general practitioner, but some hospital variants	MI	medicines information/myocardial infarction
		MR	modified release
FVC	forced vital capacity	MRC	medicines reminder chart ('compliance chart')
GDM	gestational diabetes mellitus	MMR	measles, mumps and rubella vaccination
GFR	glomerular filtration rate		
GGT	gamma-glutamyl transferase (transpeptidase)	Na^+	sodium
		NAD	nothing adverse detected
GI	gastrointestinal	NBM	'nil by mouth'
GORD	gastro-oesophageal reflux disease	NHS	National Health Service (UK)
GP	general practitioner	NICE	National Institute for Health and Clinical Excellence (England and Wales)
GTN	glyceryl trinitrate		
HAQ	Health Activity Questionnaire		
Hb	haemoglobin	NKDA	no known drug allergies
HbA_{1c}	glycated haemoglobin (marker of longer-term glucose concentrations)	NRT	nicotine replacement therapy
		NSAID	non-steroidal anti-inflammatory drug, e.g. ibuprofen
HCO_3^-	bicarbonate		
HDL	high-density lipoprotein	NSF	National Service Framework
HLA	human leucocyte antigen	NSTEMI	non-Q-wave myocardial infarction
HRT	hormone replacement therapy	OCP	oral contraceptive pill
IBD	inflammatory bowel disease	od	once daily
IgG	immunoglobulin G	O/E	on examination
IHD	ischaemic heart disease	OGD	oesophagogastroduodenoscopy – medical test
IL1-RA	interleukin 1 receptor antagonist		
IM	intramuscular	OGTT	oral glucose tolerance test
INR	international normalised ratio: monitors warfarin therapy	om/mane	each morning
		on/nocte	each night
IV	intravenous	OTC	'over-the-counter' (medicine)
K^+	potassium	PC	presenting complaint
K/DOQI	Kidney Dialysis Outcomes Quality Initiative (US)	PCA	patient-controlled analgesia
		PCP	*Pneumocystis carinii* pneumonia
LDL	low-density lipoprotein	PCT	primary care trust
LFT	liver function tests	PE	pulmonary embolism
LMWH	low-molecular-weight heparin	PEFR	peak expiratory flow rate
LVSD	left ventricular systolic dysfunction	PEG	percutaneous endoscopic gastrostomy

PMH	past/previous medical history	SSRI	selective serotonin reuptake inhibitor, e.g. fluoxetine
PO_4^{3-}	phosphate		
PPI	proton pump inhibitor, e.g. omeprazole	TCA	tricyclic antidepressant, e.g. amitriptyline
prn	when required	TED	thromboembolic deterrent
PTH	parathyroid hormone	TEMPO	Trial of Etanercept and Methotrexate with Radiographic Patient Outcomes
PUD	peptic ulcer disease		
PVD	peripheral vascular disease		
qds	four times a day	TPN	total parenteral nutrition (intravenous feeding)
RA	rheumatoid arthritis		
RLCCB	rate-limiting calcium channel blocker, e.g. diltiazem	tds	three times a day
		TNF-α	tumour/tissue necrosis factor alpha
ROS	review of systems	TSH	thyroid-stimulating hormone
SaO_2	arterial oxygen saturation	T_3	triiodothyronine
SBP	spontaneous bacterial peritonitis	T_4	thyroxine
SC	subcutaneous	UC	ulcerative colitis
SH or SHx	social history	U+Es	'urea and electrolytes', i.e. basic blood chemistry
SIADH	syndrome of inappropriate antidiuretic hormone secretion		
		UKPDS	United Kingdom Prospective Diabetes Study (for type 2 DM)
SIGN	Scottish Intercollegiate Guidelines Network		
		UTI	urinary tract infection
SPC	summary of product characteristics	WCC	white cell count (raised in infections and some malignancies)
SR	sustained release	WHO	World Health Organization

Index

Page numbers in *italics* refer to figures, tables and charts. Abbreviations are listed on pages 167–169.